TABLE OF CONTENTS

INTRODUCTION

A world wide epidemic of over-diagnosis and over-treatment of prostate cancer began in the United States in 1987 when the prostate specific antigen (PSA) test became available. I began a manuscript decrying the epidemic in 2002. By 2012, the US Preventive Task Force (USPTF) had ruled that the PSA test when used for screening did more harm than good, and that Medicare carriers did not have to reimburse for it. Immediately, radical prostatectomy rates began to fall. In that same year, 2012, two randomized prospective, controlled studies of radical prostatectomy reported no difference in cancer specific mortality between radical surgery and no surgery. This removed the rationale for early diagnosis with PSA because it meant that total ablation by any means would not lead to measurable prolongation of cancer specific life.

Another paradigm shift occurred when the American Cancer Society admitted that its early diagnosis campaign begun after World War II had not reduced the number of cancers that present as metastases proportionate to the amount of early discovery. True cancers that can metastasize start doing that at 2 mm, below the threshold of specificity for any screening test. In 2017, the percent of patients presenting their prostate cancer as metastases went up sharply compared to 2012 but this was because the cancer data were no longer diluted by incidental cancers of no clinical significance.

There has been a 30-40% decline in radical prostatectomies, 2012-2014, in areas of the country that voted for Hillary Clinton (e.g. certain practices in New York City). There has been only a 3% decline in my area of the country, the southern San Joaquin Valley, when 2012 is compared to 2014. My valley went for President Trump with the exception of the three college town of Fresno. A national hospital based figure reported at the American Urological Association (AUA) meeting in April 2018 in San Francisco, which combined both high and low utilization areas, showed a 9.01% decrease for standard 'open' radical prostatectomy rates while robot assisted radical prostatectomy declined 8.6%. Both have held level for 2014-2015. This contrasts with another national study of nine high volume centers with longer follow-up which showed a 22.6% decline in surgical volume when 2008-2012 is compared to 2012-2016. At the same AUA 2018 meeting, drastic socioeconomic differences in radical prostatectomy utilization were found in the data in the New York State Statewide Planning and Research Cooperative system.

The epidemic of over-diagnosis and over-treatment is moderating as a result of USPTF but it is far from over in 2018. It is dismaying to see the epidemic 'picking up steam' in the developing world such as the Philippines. It is the purpose of this new edition to spare the rest of the world the ravages of incontinence, impotence, depression, suicide, post-op deaths, and expense that follow radical prostatectomy or radiation for putative cure without a level 1 series showing significant life extension for either.

EXECUTIVE SUMMARY

What have our citizens bought in the United States prostate cancer pit, as noisy as the real pits at the Chicago Board of Trade? One answer is 2,800 extra deaths within 30 days of radical prostatectomy in the United States between 1985 and 1997. Every graph of prostate cancer mortality in the developed world shows a sudden upsurge in 1987-1989 immediately after prostate specific antigen testing (PSA) was introduced. Similarly there is an abrupt fall in mortality from a peak in 1995. These were the years that the radical cancer surgery rate peaked in the Medicare population in men over age 75. These deaths were the visible 'iceberg' signaling a far greater number of operative complications such as cognitive impairment in the elderly caused by low blood pressure and anemia, shortening of the penis by two centimeters, impotence, loss of libido, urinary incontinence with and without orgasm, bladder neck contracture, suicidal depression, rectal burns, as well as radiation induced killer cancers of the bladder, prostate, and rectum.

I do not call the victims of this epidemic, when they first present, patients. That word comes from the Latin, patiens, the present past participle of patior, to suffer, to endure. These men did not come to the urologist's office suffering the symptoms of prostate cancer. Most have come because of elevations of prostate specific antigen (PSA) in their blood. Others came with symptoms of benign prostatic hypertrophy (BPH). BPH caused the 'elevations' of PSA, not cancer. But BPH and prostate cancer start at the same time and develop at almost parallel rates as the result of a third variable, age. The occult, incidental cancers whose radical, wide excision caused the deaths and complications noted above were found serendipitously when the PSA elevations caused by the BPH were followed up by needle biopsies. Only one in 360 non-palpable cancers in men over 50 causes death.

After the World War II Nuremberg medical trials, animal models were considered a mandatory prelude to the introduction of any new, dangerous, medical, surgical, or radiation treatment for humans. But, no animal models in regard to radical surgery and radiation for prostate cancer have ever been published which satisfy the Nuremberg criteria. The developed world has experimented on human prostate cancer as though we had learned nothing from the Nazis.

How could a society that achieved success in World War II through science and then rededicated itself to science in the Sputnik era allow an epidemic of unscientific

3

treatments based on a religious enthusiasm to restart in the late 1970s and continue to the present day? The historian, Francis Fukuyama, identified a worldwide revolt in the 1960s against all kinds of hierarchies, including that of formal science which he called "the great disruption." Ludmerer, a historian of medical education, echoed him by noting the disappearance of hats from men and white gloves from women. This erasure of signs of status was caused by the "information revolution" according to Fukuyama. If everybody including the janitor can find on the internet aggregate data previously available only to a full professor or a CEO, then everybody can be an expert on any topic, including prostate cancer. So goes Fukuyama's argument.

In the universities, science as practiced by Condourcet, Benjamin Franklin, and Newton, was assaulted by the French deconstructionists, themselves a product of the French student riots of 1968. They said words had no fixed meaning and that therefore science with its attendant hierarchies was impossible. Their ideas were rejected by the old universities of Europe and England as a justification of propaganda, but found fertile ground at Johns Hopkins in Maryland. From there, the anti-science of French literary deconstruction infected many of the newer universities in the American West and at least one department of urology. I began my residency in urology in an "old world" which was not "brave" in the summer of 1969 at the Columbia Presbyterian Hospital and Vanderbilt Clinic on Washington Heights in New York City. There, the proper diagnosis and therapy for prostate cancer care had been determined by an intact hierarchy in the Northeast and Chicago that believed that scientific truth exists, mostly in English, on paper, independent of personal power. A brief post-war frenzy of radiotherapy and radical surgery had come and gone, discredited by hard science written by these same people. Like Jimmy Hoffa, radiotherapy and radical surgery had disappeared. Urology on the Washington heights had not yet been affected by the Fukuyama's "Great Disruption" even though, 25 minutes downtown by the A train to Wall Street, white gloves and hats were fast disappearing. The editor of the Journal of Urology, John Grayhack, M.D., upheld Abraham Flexner's full-time ideal at the University of Chicago medical school. Another Chicago full-timer, Charles Huggins, had won the Nobel Prize in 1942 for a systemic therapy for prostate cancer, androgen deprivation. The word, cure, was not allowed in the Journal of Urology in reference to prostate cancer while it was edited by Dr. Grayhack. In 1973, the year of my chief residency in urology at Columbia Presbyterian, the Journal of Urology had my first published medical article, but did not have a single one about radical prostatectomy.

The demise of the radical and radiation was not for a lack of aggression in the men of World War II when they returned to academia. Robert Lich, M.D., Professor and Chairman of Urology at the University of Louisville in Kentucky 1947-1973, introduced the British approach to the prostate from above instead of the Maryland approach from the bottom. But his claims of cure foundered on the fact that the occult cancers to be found at autopsy far outnumbered the prostate cancer deaths in a year. Data had been published in the 1960s which showed that persons with incidental carcinomas discovered in the fragments removed during transurethral operations for benign prostatic enlargement (BPH) had survival curves indistinguishable from the general population. To his credit, Dr. Lich abandoned his claims of cure when two patients returned to his office dying of prostate cancer 27 years after apparently curative operations. He advised his successor Mohammed Amin, M.D., to stay away from the procedure.

It was also common knowledge in 1973 that this cancer metastasized before it was palpable. Pre-war pathologists had observed in the late 1930s that metastases to the lymphatics around the nerves in the prostate could be identified near the smallest, incidental cancers discovered at autopsy. The harder one looked the more metastases one found. Radiation had also been discredited not only because the disease was systemic at the time of diagnosis, but also because this cancer was insensitive to radiation. We residents said these things like prayers in our weekly clinical conferences.

We did not deceive the patients in those days by claiming that there was a capsule, as impervious as Saran wrap that kept the cancer cells confined. Second year medical students knew that metastases from this kind of cancer floated away via lymphatics and the veins, not by burrowing out through the prostate capsule like some kind of shipworm. We required these cancers to be either palpable or to show an associated elevation in the blood of a marker of prostate cancer called prostatic acid phosphatase for the cancer to be significant. When this occurred, the proper treatment was believed to be systemic namely, deprivation of male hormone. Only two attendings at the Columbia Presbyterian Hospital in New York persisted in attempts at cure with radical prostatectomy. When they did it, they were considered low life by some of us.

To rule out distant spread prior to the radical surgery, we drew samples of prostatic acid phosphatase from the circulating blood and from the bone marrow prior to a proposed radical prostatectomy. When the prostatic acid phosphatase level in the bone marrow was higher than in the peripheral blood, radical surgery was cancelled and hormone deprivation was offered to the patient. Information from a bone marrow aspirate was studied because of the known affinity of this cancer for marrow. Radiation was no longer offered. We did not ask the patient for his opinion on these matters.

I recall a moment in 1973, when the systemic, non-focal paradigm for prostate cancer began to unravel in my department. John K. Lattimer, M.D., chairman of the Department of Urology and the president of the American Urological Association at the time, told us that a new radiation technique of supervoltage was being started at Stanford by Malcolm Bagshaw. He said, "Nobody knows what the effect will be of radiation on the bleeding shell" left after the old open enucleation of benign prostatic hypertrophy or after the new transurethral resection which contained an incidental, occult cancer. In fact, everybody who had studied the biology of radiation at that time knew that prostate cancer was radiation resistant and that failure of radiation was caused by the metastatic nature of the cancer. Neveretheless, Cornelius Ryan, author of *The Longest Day* and *A Bridge Too Far*, flew out to Stanford that year to see if supervoltage to the primary site of his own cancer might stop it. He elected radioactive seeds at Memorial Sloan Kettering in New York, another discredited radiation technique, and died an accelerated death.

When I left a solo private practice in Manhattan to join a the new Marshall School of Medicine in Huntington West Virginia in 1983, there had been a series of papers published by urologists documenting the increased nuclear disorganization and persistence of cancer cells in the prostate after supervoltage. After my arrival at the medical school, Michael Seddon, M.D., the Canadian trained chief of the section of Urology, stopped all referrals of prostate cancer from the local Veterans Administration Hospital to a local private practice in radiotherapy.

Radical prostatectomies by the medical school faculty also stopped because (1) Dr. Seddon did not believe in them and (2) I replaced the man who was doing them.

Alas, supervoltage radiotherapy thrived like a weed elsewhere. In my opinion, it was the rising fashion of supervoltage radiation, with its imputations of cure via focal treatment to the primary site that facilitated, the re-introduction in 1983, of the exiled, disgraced, radical prostatectomy. The radical returned as, what I call in urologic gatherings, a total, simple prostatectomy. Radical, in medical jargon, means that all the adjacent tissues are taken with the cancer. Simple means the organ is shelled out of its bed, leaving adjacent tissues. This is the new version of the old operation as described by Patrick Walsh, M.D., of Johns Hopkins. In this operation, the prostate with its capsule was shelled out of the adjacent fat as a way to spare the nerves to the voluntary gate muscle of the bladder, the penile arteries, and veins. Dr. Walsh's papers written in support of this operation never offered a new oncologic hypothesis to contest the older, established view that all these cancers were metastatic at the time of discovery. The lack of proof of concept did not matter in the ensuing market bubble. The return of the word cure to the urologist's vocabulary appealed to the action oriented, insured, middle classes of the United States.

Old money did not take the bait so eagerly. The northeast of the United States, an even more precise example is the posh northwest corner of Connecticut, and pricey, sophisticated areas of the far west like San Francisco, eschewed the revived operation. The docs in these areas did not think much of the resuscitation of William Halsted's nineteenth century hypothesis, *i.e.* that failure via metastases after local of excision of an intrinsically metastatic cancer was caused by insufficiently wide surgical margins around the primary site. To reassert this canard was an insult to the old University of Chicago, Harvard, and Columbia power structure. I spoke for this older hierarchy when I asked Patrick Walsh, M.D., chairman of Urology at Johns Hopkins, at the meeting of the mid-Atlantic section of the American Urological Association in 1984 how he reconciled his claim of cure with the 1/380 ratio of prostate cancer deaths to autopsy prevalence published the previous year in a monograph by Thomas Stamey, Professor of Urology at Stanford. He replied that one third of men who present to urologists with symptoms of prostate cancer die of it. He and everybody in the room knew that the patients he was operating upon were not presenting with symptoms of cancer. They were presenting with symptoms of benign prostatic hypertrophy (BPH). The cancers were incidental and occult at the edge of the large benign smooth muscle tumors. His answer was evasive.

The revival of the idea of cure in its plain meaning by radical prostatectomy or radiation was not caused directly by the medical schools. It was caused by the Association of Medical Schools with hospitals mandated by Abraham Flexner in 1910. Unfortunately for the United States citizens, the hospitals had become addicted to the Medicare/Medicaid money which started to flow their way in 1965.

But, in 1983, the year of Dr. Walsh's re-introduction of the total, simple prostatectomy, Medicare changed its reimbursement to "diagnostic related groups," the dreaded DRG. This meant that no matter how many days the patient stayed in the hospital or how many diagnostic tests were ordered, the hospitals got the same amount of money. It was no longer a cost + small profit proposition. A sharp contraction of revenue ensued, and the Johns Hopkins Hospital, along with all the other nineteenth century, central city, non-profit U.S. hospitals was threatened with bankruptcy. Since the medical school owned the hospital, an uncommon arrangement, the medical school was threatened by a business issue. The revenues generated by Dr. Walsh's patients helped save the hospital and the school.

Professor Fukuyama predicts oscillations toward order from disorderly periods of history *e.g.* the 1960s. This has occurred in the world of prostate cancer. The Medicare administration, the American Urological Association (1995), the Veterans Administration and a British Working Party all completed meta-analyses of the literature of total prostatectomy and radiation for scientific evidence of cancer specific life extension in the 1990s. They did not find it for either treatment. Even in 2012 such evidence does not exist.

As part of a Fukuyama like oscillation toward order, the United States has slowed its descent into an irrational abyss of screening and case finding. In March of 2009, the failure of systematic screening to prolong life was widely reported in all the popular media. The systemic paradigm characteristic of my urology residency years in New York has returned because of new data in man and animals. There has been renewed enthusiasm for androgen deprivation at an early stage. The Medicare administration has campaigned against screening and radical prostatectomy in men older than 75. In addition, a well tolerated cell poison medication, Mitoxanterone, when administered at the time of early androgen ablation has been shown in England to prolong overall survival after 10 years of follow up; a microtubule poison isolated from the yew tree may be even more effective. Drugs that prevent the growth of new blood vessels will slow this cancer. This will include aspirin or the much maligned COX-2 inhibitors such as Celebrex. Tyrosine kinase inhibitors derived from soybeans look promising. They are already proven in kidney cancer.

We will be slowing growth, not curing. No similar crescendo of evidence on a deepening, widening, experimental base has been published for surgery or radiation. I hear only the whine of wheels spinning in the mud. There has been a steady decline in radical prostatectomies as we enter the new century, the good news. The bad news is that radioactive seed implantations have surpassed radical surgery and constitute a new epidemic of radiation induced cancers.

That's the background for this book. This surgeon / specialist / journalist has been in the operating room for 58 years, 17 years under Federal Socialism, and 41 years in the private sector. Military promotion boards look for the "sound of the guns." This book has that sound. I am not a full-timer in an endowed chair. I have worked mostly in the trenches of a solo private practice tilted toward academic practice by choice. For this reason, the book respects E.O. Wilson's call for consilience, Abraham Flexner's prescription of the humanities as a tool to select priorities, and A.D. Nuthall's definition of scholarship as accuracy at the edges of the main argument.[3]

CHAPTER 1

Epidemics of over-zealous case finding and over-treatment in other cancers.

"Bernard Fisher, M.D., Distinguished Service Professor at the University of Pittsburgh is pleased to announce the withdrawal of his lawsuit against the University of Pittsburgh and the federal government in accordance with the settlement agreement that the parties reached yesterday, Release, August 27, 1997"[4]

Bernard Fisher, M.D., lost his job and his full professorship at the University of Pittsburgh because he showed that radical mastectomy, resection of the breast, nearby uninvolved muscles, and lymph nodes, for true breast cancer was no better than lumpectomy in regard to cancer control. His proof that the lesser procedure gave the same results as a big procedure threatened all those in the universities who did the big procedure for a livelihood and all those who lived in constant pain because they had given consent for an unproven operation. The latter felt like fools who had fallen for a remunerative trick. Dr. Fisher sued the federal government and collected 2.5 million in a settlement three days before going to trial. He got a formal letter of apology. This was the last shot in the "Breast Cancer Wars" 1940-1997 of which Barron Lerner's book is an eloquent account.

Despite the ministrations of an army of surgeons and mammographers, the graph of the breast cancer death rate per hundred thousand published every year by the American Cancer Society is almost level from 1930 to the present day. A slight decline in the last four years has been caused, not by earlier discovery and focal surgery, but by earlier systemic treatment, with tamoxiphen, the aromatase inhibitors,[5] and chemotherapy when used early. Despite the lack of a prospective, randomized, controlled trial during the 65 years preceding my medical school days, Halstead's late nineteenth century radical mastectomy idea persisted into the early 1960s. To me and to the other students, even then, this operation appeared to be more suitable to a *tableau vivant* at colonial

Williamsburg or Thomas Eakins's painting, *The Anatomy Lesson*. We had learned from the pathology department the year before that the true killer breast cancers, not the intraductal and/or lobular carcinomata in situ which represent 1/3 of the neoplasms discovered by mammography and present in 20% of female autopsies[6], had inevitably spread throughout the body at the time of discovery. Judah Folkman and his collaborators/competitors tell us now that the crucial volume that excites new blood vessels and the resulting metastasis is a diameter of two millimeters, below the threshold of specificity, *i.e.* 80% true positives, for mammography by MRI, ultrasound, conventional X-ray, or any blood test. By the third year surgery rotation we were supposed to have forgotten what the Department of Pathology had taught us and to believe that removing uninvolved muscles of the chest was going to improve survival. We were supposed to be impressed by Cushman Haagenson, M.D., a pathologist without a surgical residency who had surgical privileges at Columbia Presbyterian Hospital for this one operation. He brought well insured patients to the medical center. Wearing his pathologist's hat, he had published a book, *Diseases of the Breast*, but we students were not impressed.

I was more impressed by Hugh Auchincloss, Jr., who, after studying his father's lack of oncologic success with the radical mastectomy since the 1930s, was pioneering, with George Crile, Jr., of the Cleveland Clinic, a modified radical mastectomy that spared women their chest muscles. Rachel Carson, author of *Silent Spring*, had such a limited resection, a lumpectomy, by Dr. Crile. By the mid-1960s Dr. Haagenson's livelihood was threatened. The results of the lesser procedure were clearly the same when compared to the radical procedure. I told a resident in general surgery in 1965 what Dr. Auchincloss was doing. The resident shot back "but he does not do it here. He does it in New Jersey" as if where he did it would change the cancer's course.

Dr. Auchincloss, who had been my preceptor in General Surgery, told me a decade later at dinner in the Century Club in New York that 'they' presumably including Cushman Haagenson had kicked him out of the Vanderbilt Clinic Breast Service at Columbia. Years later in the 1990s, I was visiting a rural hospital in Arkansas and was told by a general surgeon that he did the Auchincloss procedure. The radical resection of the chest muscles that had been presented as life saving by Professor Haagenson in New York City in the 1960s had been discarded in the Ozarks by the 1980s. Even so, in 1992, only about ten percent of mastectomies in the western United States were "lumpectomies." Dr. Fischer had not yet won his 1997 settlement for two and a half million from the federal government.

The value of a 'lumpectomy' is to diagnose the cancer, to divine prognosis by its look under the microscope and encourage early systemic therapy if it is clearly metastatic. Systemic therapy has prolonged life slightly in the past four years. The improvements in "mortality" that are touted by the American Cancer Society's report every year to encourage early diagnosis[7] turn out to be only improved five year survival. Ten years survival data is the minimum for breast cancer data to be credible in private practice.[8] Some women, like the infamous judge Rose Byrd of California, have died of breast cancer 20 years after diagnosis. The alleged improvement is ascribable to lead time bias and stage migration. See the glossary at the end of this book. Women transformed into "patients" by mammograms know for a longer time that they have a bad cancer but they die at the time appointed by net of the mitotic rate minus the cell suicide rate, the "doubling time." DNA is destiny. The ten year survival data shows only slight improvement at high cost.

Breast cancer doubling times are variable. They range from 44 to 1869 days.[9] On average, breast cells divide more frequently than prostate cancer cells. Their mean doubling time has been measured to be 212 days[10] about twice as fast as prostate cancer's mean of 475 days (380 to 570). Theoretically, using the 212 doubling time, it should take 16^{11}, instead of 39 years in the case of prostate cancer[12], for an average breast cancer to reach the one centimeter size detectable with reasonable specificity (80%) by mammograms. It takes four years for a breast cancer tumor to grow from two millimeters to one centimeter. One centimeter is the minimum for an image to have specificity for a cancer diagnosis. Therefore, four years of metastases have occurred before mammography can discover a cancer. Mammography is never "in time" to prevent metastases. The total duration of a breast cancer from the error in DNA replication that allows metastases to thrive to death ranges from 7 to 25 years, instead of the 52 years for prostate cancer.

As in the case of incidental, occult non-fatal prostate cancers, the pro-screening, pro-surgery publicists in breast cancer have created an epidemic of lobular carcinoma in situ,[13] a pre-cancer. Lobular carcinoma in situ is an "observation," not an illness. It sounds ominous that one retrospective series reported a 50% rate of invasive cancers found in selected women with carcinoma in situ placed on surveillance.[14] But that is retrospective. The critical data point, the proportion of lobular carcinomata in situ that are subject to further errors in the DNA that allow metastases to thrive cancers is unknown. We have no 'denominator' to this fraction. It is because of the increased discovery of the denominator, the pre-cancers, without knowledge of the numerator, metastasizing cancers derived from the pre-cancers, that selling mammography machines is profitable for General Electric. For example, a recent United States Secretary of Agriculture was "cured" of lobular carcinoma in situ.

Large sums of money are circulating on this shaky ground. Some radiologists do nothing but mammograms for a living. Some lawyers make a living suing them for "missing" cancers. For that reason, radiologists over-interpret an image that is not specific. They order more mammograms and more cancer causing radiation. They suggest biopsies by a surgeon or do it themselves with a needle and pay, thereby, medical school debts, mortgages, and college tuitions for their children. Drug companies make money with gene tests.[15] It is taking money from the worried well, which would include those with pre-cancers, that provides the best marginal return on capital for the individual practitioner. For institutions, it is the facility fee. True patients, sufferers with symptomatic metastases do not compete well, as a business proposition, with those who have none.

As is true for prostate cancer, bone marrow aspirations for cytokeratin-positive cells using immuno-cytochemical techniques unmask the pretense that breast cancer can be chopped out "in time" to prevent metastases. For example, 199 of 552 patients (36%) who had been operated upon for breast cancer for alleged "cure" had cancer cells in their marrow on the day of operation.[16] *Aficionados* of local excision typically cry out, "No correlation with clinical deterioration has been proved!" This is a false statement. Bone marrow positivity has been correlated with clinical deterioration and death from breast cancer with as little as four years follow-up.[17] The authors of this study cautioned that, in breast cancer, a minimum of 10 to 15 years is necessary to make a comment about the presence or absence of metastases.[18] These intervals sound like prostate cancer[19] and they tell us why the claims of the American Cancer Society of progress against true breast cancer through early discovery and focal removal are false. This same correlation of bone marrows positive for cytokeratin with clinical deterioration has been found for colorectal cancer,[20] gastric,[21] and non-small-cell lung carcinoma.[22]

Consider the thyroid cancer industry. The sporadic adult, as opposed to the hereditary form found in juveniles,[23] well differentiated thyroid cancer is present in 22 percent of autopsies when immuno-cytochemical stainings are used.[24] Over the whole population of the United States, that represents millions. Twenty-two percent of your friends and neighbors are not dying of thyroid cancer. In fact, during my six years of residency in university hospitals in New York City, I never came near to (or even heard about) a patient dying of thyroid cancer in those hospitals. I have not encountered one instance of such a death in other settings in the 35 years since. The closest I have come to a thyroid cancer death has been to read about Max Lerner's daughter (see the chapter on humanists) and William Rehnquist, a deceased chief justice of the Supreme Court. Only one out of 450 persons with the incidental, well differentiated, adult thyroid cancer becomes symptomatic.[25] This ratio is even smaller than the drastically small ratio of one death from prostate cancer to 380 prostate cancers present at autopsy. And yet there are M.D.s earning a living generating survivors of this clinically insignificant cancer. By contrast, the ratio of pancreatic cancers which cause death to incidental pancreatic cancers found at autopsy is 1/1.2. Pancreatic cancer killed Luciano Pavarroti, the great tenor, in one year. The five year survival rate for pancreatic cancer is currently 4% in all races as compared to thyroid cancer's 96% and prostate's 98%. Pancreatic cancer is what every man thinks of when he/she uses the word "cancer." It is insincere of the cancer industry to advertise for patients with clinically insignificant cancers without notifying the public that the industry has taken the hawsers off the mooring of the 'plain meaning' of the word cancer.

The most vivid example of how a cancer screening program may be a disaster is the story of a urine test for neuroblastoma, an uncommon cancer of childhood. This urine test was used to screen infants at three and six months in Quebec.[26] The controls were an **unscreened** population in the U.S. There was no improvement in the death rate of the screened children. Even worse, 19 of the 22 children who died had been screened with negative results because their cancer had ceased to make the chemicals detected in urine. The worst prostate cancers, the reader will learn in the chapter on PSA, may cease to make the screening molecule. By contrast, almost all the tumors detected by the neuroblastoma urine screening test had favorable biologic features. This meant the tumors would likely spontaneously regress, re-differentiate, the "cure" characteristic of this tumor. All these children were alive at the time of the report except two with severe complications of treatment which may have been unnecessary because of the spontaneous regression phenomenon. It is tempting to think they would have been better off with no treatment.

This was a shocking result. A German group tried to change it by screening later, at one year of age.[27] They hoped to thereby skip the tumors that would spontaneously regress but catch more of the killers. They too found no improvement in the death rate. Two thirds of all their detected cases would have regressed without clinical detection. Worse, two children detected by screening died from complications of surgery and one from too much chemotherapy. From a public health point of view, screening for this cancer was a disaster.

The analogy with prostate specific antigen (PSA) screening is close. One screens for molecules that are a unique product of the deranged cancer cell's original morphology. The problem is that many of the tumors composed of cells well enough organized to make those molecules are well enough behaved to be subject to the body's inherent controls of cell growth. They pose no threat. The killers in the neuroblastoma study were made up of poorly differentiated cells which did not make the sentinel molecule, just as poorly differentiated cancer of the prostate, (Gleason grade 8-10), makes little PSA per unit volume compared to the better looking cells. The authors of both neuroblastoma papers called for a cessation of screening. It has ceased world wide.

The broader meaning of the failure of the neuroblastoma screening program in infants was not lost on Masters of Public Health earning their living screening adults for cancer. Russell Harris, M.D., of the University of North Carolina told the New York Times that the neuroblastoma story was an example of the hazards of screening for cancer. He was reported as saying that most screening tests, including the prostate specific antigen test, were being used before they had been proven to yield an improved outcome over an unscreened population.[28] He mentioned New York-Cornell's experimental screening for lung cancer via extra sensitive computerized radiation induced images of the chest in smokers over 50. He said the results have not been compared to an unscreened population. An M.D. in private practice in Manhattan, where this lung cancer screening epidemic broke out, told me that it has created clinical chaos in the form of the discovery of small densities that might or might not be worthy of biopsy. Because of the irreducible hazards of general anesthesia, it is a sure but unadvertised bet that fatalities have occurred in New York citizens before the microscopic slides were available. Nonetheless, the week after preliminary results were published, the New York Times reported the phone was 'ringing off the hook' at the N.Y.-Cornell radiology department, the Pavlovian "reward" of any screening program.

The reader can see now that the epidemic of case finding and excess treatment subject to "push back" in this book is not the first. It has been preceded by epidemics of care in thyroid and breast cancer, neuroblastoma, colon cancer[29] and now coincides with an epidemic in the lung cancer "market." All instances except neuroblastoma in pediatrics, where there is little insurance money, have achieved a bogus respectability through lead time bias, stage migration and the "cure" of tumors that had minimal metastatic potential. These doctors caused (iatrogenic) epidemics that have created unease among those possessing the increasingly common Master of Public Health degree. The reader will learn that a similar unease was present in Michael Korda's prostate cancer support group. Ivan Ilych's *Medical Nemesis* sensed the remunerative scam. Cornelius Ryan and Anatole Broyard, two prostate cancer sufferers who were also sophisticated New Yorkers, were not impressed by their initial contacts with the industry, as the reader will see in the chapter on the humanists' response.

CHAPTER 2

Benign prostatic hypertrophy (BPH), a non-malignant tumor of the prostate that can kill you.

In the abdomen, benign tumors, such as fibroid tumors of the uterus, can grow to a large size without symptoms. But when a benign tumor's growth is confined by bone, *e.g.* the pituitary, havoc ensues. Because the boney pelvis confines the growth of benign prostatic hypertrophy (BPH), it pushes inward toward the urethra. The pressures developed by the bladder muscle to cause urination are very low, the weight of a 60 centimeter column of water, nowhere near blood pressure values. This means that a small increase in resistance to urinary flow caused by encroaching BPH can cause the incomplete emptying noted by men as double voiding. True sufferers from BPH, not "socially constructed" patients, void and five minutes later want to void again. They are just taking the "top" off the reservoir of urine. In a functional sense, their storage volume has become much smaller. They are up all night.

The prostate specific antigen test, PSA, introduced in 1987, has made millions for Abbot Labs. It has excellent specificity for BPH at action values between 4 and 10ug/cc[30] but is a little advertised dud in regard to specificity for prostate cancer at those same action values. Despite its lousy specificity, the PSA blood test has triggered an enormous number of prostate biopsies because of a value greater than 4.0 ug/cc in the period 1987-2009. This error in the assessment of the prospective probabilities by United States M.D.s in private practice caused, in turn, a world wide epidemic of radiation and radical surgery injuries, the subject of this book.

Benign prostatic hypertrophy (BPH) starts as an over production of smooth muscle (rather like a woman's fibroid tumor) at age thirty to forty in the area next to the urethra. Cancer begins in the outermost rim at the same time. The two pathologies are not related. See Figure 1. Some think a substance comes up the vas deferens from the testis to inspire this proliferation. It could be an extra dose of male hormone in the lumen of the vas deferens.

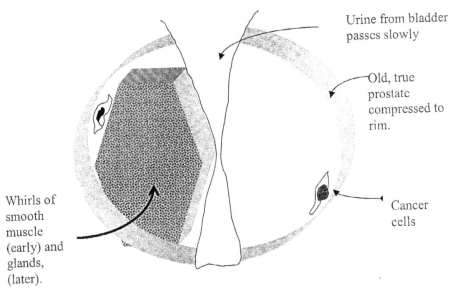

Urine from bladder
passes slowly

Old, true
prostate
compressed to
rim.

Cancer
cells

Whirls of
smooth
muscle
(early) and
glands,
(later).

FIGURE 1

The multiplication of benign smooth muscle cells begins about age 40 in 30% of men. Only later, after age 60, do the glandular cells which make PSA begin to predominate. The ducts that carry the prostatic fluid with its PSA are then obstructed by lateral pressure from the growing whorls of BPH. This causes the PSA to leak into the blood stream. Also, bacterial contamination of the BPH causes inflammation and subsequent stricture of the six ducts that connect to the urethra. This causes the false positive 'elevations' of PSA. The 'action value' for PSA was set far too low at 4ug/dl.

BPH has a 30% incidence of cancer of its own.[31] These cancers start in a younger DNA with less drastic errors and therefore seldom kill. The enthusiasts for radical surgery and/or radiation with intent to cure claim that they are not operating on these incidental non-killers. For this argument to prevail, the major series of radical prostatectomies and radiotherapy for "cure" would have to say in their "methods" section that they have excluded the cancers that arise from B.P.H., that they are only operating on "rim" cancers from the compressed true prostate as seen in Figure 1. I do not find such statements in the literature. Moreover, transurethral resection of BPH[32] means, in my hands, a finger in a rectal sheath for palpation of the cutting loop at all times.[33] The resection should always be taken out to the compressed, older periphery where the more virulent cancers lurk. Transurethral resection in experienced hands always samples the cancer prone, peripheral true prostate. It discovers the same population of cancers as those discovered by transrectal ultrasound guided biopsy. See the chapter on this technique. The reader needs to know all this because, during the peak of the epidemic of 1992-1994, a 32% drop in the frequency of operations appropriate for BPH in 1992[34] suggested that in some areas of the United States radical surgery for cancer had been substituted for the operations appropriate for BPH. I saw an example of that substitution at the Minneapolis Veterans Administration clinic.

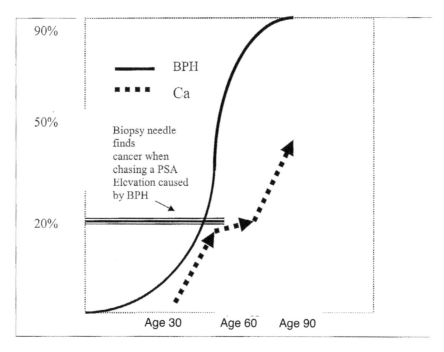

FIGURE 2

Both BPH and cancer develop in parallel from ages 30 to 50. 30% of the cancers develop in BPH, but they are well differentiated, not killers. Biopsies provoked by an 'elevated' PSA due to BPH discover the 20-30% of occult cancers present in autopsies of men 50-60 years old. This is identical to the 30% pitifully low, positive rate for PSA alone as a screening tool. No more cancers have been discovered in the PSA era than would have been found in a random series of men that age off the street whose PSA was unknown.

The early, younger than age sixty, smooth muscle phase of obstruction by BPH can be successfully palliated by pharmacologic blockade of the sympathetic amines, the fight-or-flight molecules, but not without a price. Blocking these molecules can lead to low blood pressure. One of my colleagues told me that his prescription of one of these drugs to a roofer almost caused the roofer to fall off a roof due to faintness on a hot day. One of my patients on this pill fainted and fell into a river with a rapid current while fishing. A second disadvantage is the cost, $30.00 a month in the private sector with a prescription medicine insurance rider, $90.00 without insurance in Wyoming. This is a prohibitive bite out of those on a fixed income, mostly social security.

This early, medical phase of BPH can also be treated by cutting furrows with a needle-like electrode through the smooth muscle bundles wrapped around the urethra in four quadrants. I did not offer this transurethral incision technique often enough to the veterans when I worked for them in a socialist system. It is underutilized in private practice as well. Microwaving in the office works well here.

In the sixth and seventh decade of life, glandular proliferation begins to predominate over smooth muscle proliferation, again proceeding outward and away from the urethra. These glands have no exit. They are obstructed, and so the prostate specific antigen (PSA) they make, a normal component of semen, is pushed into the blood by rising intraductal pressure. The ducts also close off as a result of compression by the smooth muscle component near the urethra. Thus, the PSA correlates with larger and larger volumes of BPH. This is clearly stated in Stamey *et al*'s seminal paper in the New England Journal of Medicine of October 8, 1987. PSA also correlates significantly with age. This age correlation is seldom mentioned in journal articles about PSA and prostate cancer. Figure 3 shows the rise of the PSA value with the volume of BPH at age forty and seventy.

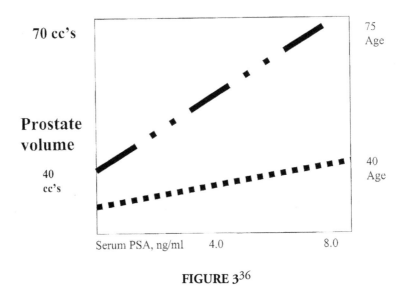

FIGURE 3[36]

A 40-year-old man with 45 ccs of BPH may have a PSA of 4.0 and not have cancer. A 75-year-old man with 70ccs of BPH is normally expected to have a PSA of 8. He would also be expected to have a 40% incidence of occult prostate cancers, four different ones on average. This is why persons with so-called elevations of PSA > 4 ng per ml. caused by BPH lose their entire prostates or are irradiated for a fictional 'cure.' If the action value had been set at 10 ng per ml. as it was in one early series,[37] hundreds of lives and millions of erections could have been saved.

The method of measurement of the volume of these large glands has been determined by the best way to insure profits for business, not by science. The concentration of PSA (micrograms per deciliter) in the blood has not been typically presented to the general public as needing a discount for the volume of BPH.[38,39] My specialty has measured the volume of BPH with transrectal ultrasound in the office. It is not the best way because it is uncomfortable, even dangerous for some cardiac patients. By contrast, John

Frachia's group at Lennox Hill Hospital in New York has shown that an ultrasound volume of the prostate determined by placing the probe just above the pubic bone (suprapubic) to look down on the prostate is just as good as the volume obtained via the transrectal route.[40] Their work confirms work by the University of Chicago years ago. It is easy to do prostate volumes via the suprapubic route if the patient has come with a full bladder. The water transmits the ultrasound waves with little distortion. Seventy percent of urologists in the west now have office ultrasound. The only caveat in regard to suprapubic ultrasound is the nation's epidemic of obesity. The image is grainy in the obese.

After age 60, Proscar, now the generic finasteride, made by Merck becomes more effective than the fight-or-flight molecule blockers. This drug and another of its class advertised on television, dutasteride, decrease the production of dihydrotestosterone (DHT), the superactive fraction of the male hormone. The prostate that will predictably respond is mostly glands, less smooth muscle. It feels squishy with retained prostatic fluid, not firm like the muscle of your thumb. Finasteride has been shown to diminish by half the number of benign prostatic hypertrophies that have to be operated because of complete inability to urinate, about a third of all BPH patients prior to this drug. A trial of cancer prevention with this drug has been published. It appears to prevent well differentiated cancers which seldom kill but not anaplastic cancers which often do.

The disadvantage to this class of drugs is that semen volume is diminished. This means that the men feel the desire for intercourse at longer intervals. Some of their wives interpret this to mean that they have girlfriends on the side, every wife's nightmare. I always caution the men to tell their wives they do not have a girlfriend. Urologists can take advantage of the semen diminishing effect of this drug class to distinguish between an elevation of PSA due to cancer from that due to BPH. If either one of the class causes the PSA to fall to half its value in three months, many urologists feel the cancer scare is off, particularly if the volume of BPH is high.

Finally, there comes a time when neither pill separately, nor even the two together, allow a good night's sleep. The men are up four to six times at night. It is this symptom of BPH that brings them into their generalist M.D.'s office in their fifties and sixties. They really are "patients" in the Latin sense of the word. They are suffering from BPH, not cancer. It is hogwash, therefore, to write that BPH is a social construct which much of the prostate cancer business is. It cannot be made to go away by French "deconstruction." Tell that to my Veterans Administration patient who was exsanguinating from giant fragile blood vessels arching over the BPH nodules projecting into his bladder. I had to transfuse him two units before I stopped the blood from pouring out with a transurethral resection.

Such patients cause me to believe in recent years that I have been waiting too long to propose transurethral resection of the prostate, the rotorutor job. See figure 4.

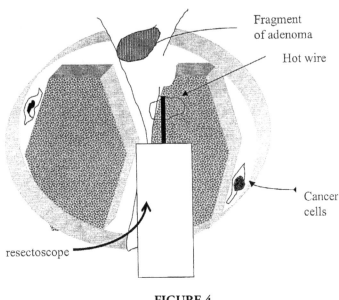

Fragment
of adenoma

Hot wire

Cancer
cells

resectoscope

FIGURE 4

The resectoscope is sent up the urethra under vision to allow whittling with a hot wire at the bilateral smooth muscle and glandular tumors. This is a transurethral resection of the prostate called by its acronym, TURP.

The problem with a long term, pill-pushing strategy is that the nodules of BPH grow to enormous size. The men get into their late eighties with one or two heart attacks before presenting legs akimbo on the operating table. In my last two years in the Veterans Administration system, I resected five instances of BPH of one hundred fifty grams or greater. I did two over 100 grams in my solo, private practice in Wyoming which followed. One of them was straight off Interstate 80. He would not stop bleeding enough for me to get him to his home six hours away in Nevada. I reported the five V.A. patients to the Western Section of the American Urological Association in 2002. I told the section that I had worked on the 250 gram monsters alternating left and right hands in two sessions of one-and-half hours each separated by one week.[41] The much higher energies, called vaporization, that we are now using for the TURP (compared to when I was trained in 1973) allow me to avoid a knife incision in the pubic crease to scoop out these tumors the size of oranges. The largest glands are mostly water because they are predominantly glandular material, not smooth muscle. It is possible to reduce them to steam, smoke, and carbon with the vaporization electrode. This technique causes less bleeding and infusion of the irrigating solution into the blood stream. I trim the smoking ruin with a thin loop. Also, pretreatment with the drugs that prevent the production of dihyrotestosterone has made these giant benign tumors less bloody during resection. Some urologists continue to use an "open" technique for these huge benign tumors but I think that is out of date.

The media's (and my specialty's) recent emphasis on prostate cancer has concealed the fact that BPH alone is a serious "plague." I remember three private patients from my Manhattan days. One was an aging intellectual on the lower west side who had all kinds of alternative theories about health and physiology. By the time I got to him, both kidneys were barely functioning shells. I had to put tubes in both his kidneys before I worked on his prostate. In that distant time before ultrasound or fluoroscopic guidance of needles, tubes meant large incisions in both flanks. The second patient was the most important admitting internist M.D. to my "flagship" hospital, St. Clare's. He had been watching the level of urea in his blood. When it rose to a level called renal 'insufficiency,' he consulted me. His ureters were the size of my wrists. I had over one thousand grams of BPH in "the bucket" after I finished his "rotorutor" job. This was preposterously large for those times. I stumbled into it because this was before we had ultrasound to properly size BPH. He had no major complications, only an infection in his big baggy ureters with a minor league bacteria called staphylococcus albus. These instances of giant BPH often call for a blood transfusion with the attendant viral dangers of hepatitis B, C, AIDS, and, now, prions.

Here is a third patient who illustrates how BPH can send you across the river Styx. I was called via my membership in the New York County Medical Society to a Manhattan medical panel which empowered to screen out worthless lawsuits. The patient in question had stepped on his catheter in the dark of the night in his postoperative period and pulled his catheter into his urethra. The balloon of the catheter split open the capsule of the prostate and caused violent bleeding. His urologist, who had been one of my instructors at Columbia Presbyterian, took him back to the operating room. He died postoperatively from the irreducible, cardiovascular reasons the elderly will die from multiple operations done close together in time. The blood thickens and clots in the coronary arteries or veins of the legs. The judge and the lawyer wanted me to hang my colleague in private practice. I refused. I said this catheter accident was part of the irreducible risk of major surgery. Benign prostatic hypertrophy and, particularly, open intracavitary surgery are inherently dangerous. The judge and lawyer were incensed at me. They wanted to set up a phony standard of care that said that major intracavitary surgery is inherently safe and only malpractice causes death. This legal theory is candy for ambulance chasers but is not true.

Lastly, it should be noted here that there are many minimal, non-cutting, surgical treatments now competing in the BPH market. They are all various forms of energy which 'cook' the cells. I am not against them for small volumes of BPH provided no attempt is made to project the energy or lack thereof (freezing) into or outside the capsule. In fact I have begun to use microwave in the office after 15 years of observing it from afar. This is for small symptomatic BPH without a middle lobe projection into the bladder. As above, I believe we should address BPH earlier than we do and not fool around with pills so long. A peak flow rate below ten cubic centimeters per second with a pre-voiding volume of two hundred and fifty cubic centimeters is a reasonable action point.[42] When the BPH is below fifty cubic centimeters, almost any of the minimal modalities, *e.g.* ultrasound, microwave, or circulating hot water, ferromagnetic thermal ablation will reduce symptoms, but not to the same refreshing degree as transurethral resection. Above sixty cubic centimeters in my opinion or with a prominent middle lobe, you have to start scooping out substance to get a satisfying symptomatic result. Medicare allowed a $650 price for this operation in 2005 in Wyoming. This is down from $1200, thirty years ago in Manhattan, and $850 in 2000. However the buying power of the dollar due to inflation caused by both political parties is about 1/3 what it was in 1975. And so I was getting about $147.00 (1973) in buying power, less than I would pay a mechanic to fix a major item in my car. This may explain the substitution of the more remunerative radical prostatectomy for transurethral resection that occurred in some areas of the country as will be detailed in the chapter on geographic anomalies in utilization.

As noted by Albarrans in the nineteenth century, quoted by Hugh Young in his 1910 paper on the first radical prostatectomies, and illustrated by figure 1, about 10% of BPH patients will have carcinomata of varying degrees of differentiation found in the "chips." Another 20% can be discovered by special stains. The rest of this book is about the epidemic of care for prostate cancer which grew out of the fad for diagnosing cancer in persons whose prostate specific antigen, PSA had been elevated by BPH and its attendant prostatitis.

CHAPTER 3

The advent of prostate specific antigen (PSA) testing; its lack of specificity.

"The elevation in PSA that accompanies the hyperplasia (.3ng per milliliter per gram of prostate tissue) precludes the use of PSA concentration as a means of screening for prostate cancer." Stamey *et al*, 1987[43]

U.S. Panel Says No to Prostate Screening for Healthy Men. "Healthy men should no longer receive a P.S.A. blood test to screen for prostate cancer because the test does not save lives overall and often leads to more tests and treatments that needlessly cause pain, impotence and incontinence in many, a key government health panel has decided."[44] Gardiner Harris, New York Times, October 6, 2011.

P SA was "gospel" according to a New York Times reporter[45] but never to all urologists; they have long had misgivings about PSA screening for prostate cancer.[46] It is the lay public, not the docs, that explains the hullabaloo that broke lose in 2001 in the San Francisco Chronicle when "…Michael Wilkes and Gavin Yamey, then editors of the Western Journal of Medicine, argued that there was no good evidence to screen healthy men for prostate cancer with the PSA test."[47] The Chronicle said they had never published a more controversial piece.[48] The lobby for screening aimed its heavy guns at Wilkes and Yamey. The reason for the heated reaction was insecurity. Three years later, Gina Kolata of the New York Times reported that the action value for PSA level used in William Catalona's influential 1991 review in the New England Journal of Medicine (NEJ) had been adopted "just sort of arbitrarily."[49] She also shrewdly observed that this NEJ article did not report on the proportion of false positives, the test of a test. Despite this omission, the entire world has adopted PSA uncritically with the disastrous results detailed here.

An enzyme called prostatic acid phosphatase was tested as a cancer screen in the 1930s. Its use as a surrogate for the growth or shrinkage of prostate cancer in response to the removal or addition of male hormone won the 1941 Nobel prize for Charles Huggins, a urologist at the University of Chicago. However, prostatic acid phosphatase was soon discovered to have too many false positives and false negatives, just as was the case with the carcino-embryonic antigen (CEA) for colon cancer.

Prostate specific antigen (PSA), was first reported in 1979 from a publicly funded New York State hospital.[50] It is not specific for prostate. It is a normal component of breast milk and saliva. It is even made by some B-cell lymphomas, a blood cancer, as I have reported.[51] PSA dissolves coagulated semen and so liberates the spermatozoa to enter the cervix and fertilize an egg.[52] Its first application was in the forensics of rape cases. Within five years, the Hybritech group, a commercial laboratory, developed a sensitive assay for this enzyme to exploit the cancer market.

When Federal Drug Administration approval was won in 1986, I began to use PSA to measure the effect of castration on obvious metastatic prostate cancer in the V.A. hospital in Walla Walla, Washington. A year later, in 1987, an article in the New England Journal of Medicine about PSA[53] by Thomas Stamey, M.D. of Stanford caused a sharp upturn in the number of biopsies and subsequent radical prostatectomies and radiation which peaked in 1992. If anybody had actually read the article as science, they would have noticed the author's statement that "the elevation in PSA that accompanies the hypeplasia…precludes the use of PSA concentration as a means of screening for prostate cancer."[54]

Fourteen years later, Dr. Stamey *et al* documented the lack of correlation between cancer volumes and PSA levels below 8-10 nanograms per ml.[55] When I heard the initial podium presentation of this data at the Western Section of the American Urological Association meeting in Monterey in September of 1999, I was not sure I had heard correctly. I used 'snail mail' to Dr. Stamey to clarify the matter. He "snail mailed" me back saying that when he reviewed his 1987 patient series he found it overweighted with PSA values greater than ten.[56] Since only values over 10 nanograms per milliliter even begin to correlate with cancer, he now realized that he had biased the interpretation of the test results by manipulating the "prospective probabilities." See the glossary. An over estimation of the discriminatory power resulted. Paul H. Lange, M.D., chairman of urology at the Universtiy of Washington, who originally testified about the usefulness of 4 ug/ml as an action value before the FDA, has endorsed Dr. Stamey's retraction of the significance of values below 10 ug/ml.[57] Non-specificity below 10 ng/ml was confirmed by a report from Europe at the 2003 annual meeting of the American Urological Association.[58]

These statements might have been King Canute railing against the waves. Physicians other than urologists proved to be a good market for a blood test for prostate cancer. Nobody likes to do rectal exams. Some internists bought machines to do the test for profit in their offices. The number of PSA tests ordered for screening purposes by non-urologists, doubled between 1991 to 1996 in the Medicare population.[59] In a younger, working age population at Kaiser Permanente, the tests per one thousand enrollees increased sixteen times from 1989 to 1996, with a brief decrease in slope after a warning by the Medicare "watch-dog" group in 1993.

Years after its adoption world wide, PSA was finally subjected to the tests of its discriminatory power that should have been required for FDA approval. The usual test of a test is a graph of sensitivity versus the specificity as seen in Figure 1. For a test to be useful, the plot of sensitivity versus specificity must curve steeply toward the upper left-hand corner. When plot of the values is simply the diagonal between the two corners, it means that as fast as you gain sensitivity and catch all the cancers you lose specificity. This means you gain an equal number of false positives. False positives are expensive. A publication about serum proteomics patterns as an improvement over the PSA test "leaks" the sad result, which was obtained from a sample with *unbiased prospective probabilities*, that the plot of sensitivity versus specificity for stand-alone PSA is the dreaded straight diagonal.[60] You could flip a coin and predict the presence or absence of cancer just as well.

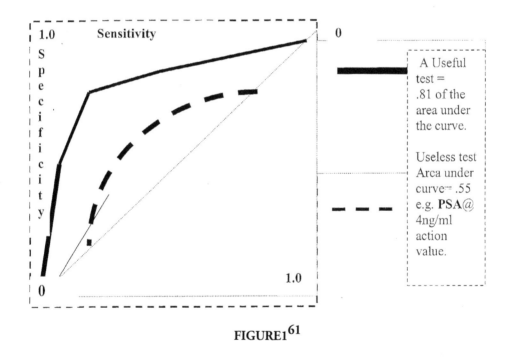

FIGURE1[61]

The test of a test is the receiver-operator curve, a graph of how specificity changes as sensitivity changes. Convention states that a test with 80% of the area under its curve is a good test. The 50% level, the small dotted line above, means the test has no discriminatory power. The area under the curve for PSA with an action value of 4.0 ug/ml is 55% in a normally distributed population over 50 years old. Thus, an elevation of PSA from 4.0 to 10 is meaningless.

There have been many attempts to fix PSAs inability to discriminate between BPH/prostatitis and cancer. For example, one group improved the discrimination of PSA by grouping men who consented to biopsy with those who did not.[62] The problem with this 'fix' is that the men who consented to a biopsy were on average 5.4 years older than those who did not.

Their mean PSA was three times higher. The reader knows from the previous chapter that sixty percent of men aged 60 who die of other causes have occult, non-palpable prostate cancer.[63] Therefore, the older mean age of the sample, the better receiver-operator-characteristic (ROC) curve of PSA looks.[64][65] Older men have more and bigger BPH, which raises the PSA, and more and bigger incidental cancers to be found serendipitously with a biopsy. These tiny cancers are not responsible for the PSA "elevation."

Yet another attempt to improve on the wretched specificity of PSA is sold by Hybritech via Beckman/Coulter machines. It compares free PSA to protein bound PSA. At its best, when the free PSA is below 12 percent of the total PSA, four times out of ten times the test indicates cancer when, in fact, there is none, a false positive rate of 40%.[66] The maximum false positive rate for a test to be "good" is 20%. Free versus bound PSA just does not make it. For me, an M.D., even more damning is that Hybritech gives no biological explanation as to why BPH should create more complexed PSA than cancer cells.

Hybritech also attempted to improve the true positive rate with direct measurement of complexed PSA. Instead of detecting cancer in 11% of biopsies, the detection rate only rose to 20% true positives,[67] still dreadful specificity. In summary, knowing the PSA value does not increase the yield of cancer beyond that expected for the age group being tested. The countercultural truth is that PSAs below 10 correlate with BPH volume not cancer, as noted in chapter 3. In 2000, Patrick Walsh, the chairman at Johns Hopkins who revived the radical prostatectomy in 1983, wrote, "To be honest, the increased PSA in many men is not a marker of cancer but of prostatic hyperplasia."[68] By that he means BPH.

The specificity of PSA under routine conditions can be improved modestly to 29% true positives by raising the biopsy trigger point to 7 ug/ml.[69] But this is nearly twice as high as the action value of 4 ug/ml currently used by the whole world. Better specificity is achieved by converting the PSA to a density, *i.e.* dividing the serum PSA level by the volume of BPH. If a density figure of .16 ug/ml per cubic centimeter of prostate is used as a signal of the presence of cancer, a true positive rate of 50% can be achieved. This is better, but still not close to the 80% true positive indicative of a good test of any kind. Sensitivity is not necessarily good (finding all the cancers there are) since we know that 60% of men age 60-70 have microscopic prostate cancer.[70]

I have used PSA density in my practice since 1988. The objection usually raised is the added cost of the transrectal ultrasound to determine prostate volume. But the cheaper suprapubic ultrasound volume correlates closely with the transrectal view in the case of the large benign prostatic hypertrophies which elevate the PSA. I used that routinely at the

Veterans Administration Hospital in Fresno to the initial consternation of the department of radiology. They came around in time. I did the exam myself for ten years in private practice in Delano, CA. I used a PSA density derived from an ultrasound measurement successfully in a malpractice suit.

There may be differences between PSA made by prostate cancers and BPH. For example, a group in Japan has shown that "PSA from cancerous materials does not contain the lower molecular mass forms."[71] However, because of the commercial success of the PSA test, "technological freeze" has set in and this line of research is undeveloped. This is not much of a loss because as prostate cancers become more malignant, and therefore more clinically significant, they lose the ability to make PSA of any kind. Remember that the most malignant neuroblastomas in children lost their markers as described in Chapter 1.

There is a second way doctors and citizens (they are not patients yet because an elevated PSA is not a disease) can separate the "wheat from the chaff" in PSA readings: citizens with a PSA value between 4.0 and 10.00 can be given finasteride, a drug which shrinks the glandular component of BPH. If the PSA level then drops 50% and goes below 4.0 ug/dl, significant cancer is unlikely if no stoney hard nodule is felt.[72] Since prostate cancer grows slowly, a three month delay to take finasteride and remeasure the PSA test is an inexpensive, low risk approach. I have just done this with a high school classmate of mine, to his immense relief.

My personal response to the epidemic of elevated PSAs has been conditioned by the fact that I spent most of the upswing of the epidemic of prostate cancer care working on a salary for the Veterans Administration. This is a capitated, government HMO. There was no way I could biopsy all the elevated PSAs and do all the urgent operations needed by the World War II population entrusted to me as a solo practitioner most of the time. The exigencies of public sector budgetary discipline forced me to read and quote to myself the papers that would justify not biopsing all of the veterans with "elevated" PSAs. By contrast, in the private sector, where more work means more money, the bias for generalists is to earn extra money by doing the PSA test in the office and then refer all elevated PSAs to a urologist in expectation of a biopsy. Urologists themselves in a hypothetical office of three can make $19,656 in annual profit doing 150 tests per month if Medicare continues to pay $25.70 per test.[73] Each false "positive" test then can generate a profitable biopsy opportunity. Urologists in private practice are not sorry about the biopsy epidemic. Pathologists in private practice are not sorry either. Medicare pays $97.03 per biopsy core. Since some academic urologists are calling for as many as 21 biopsies, the taxpayer is looking at charges of $2037.63 per transrectal biopsy session flowing into pathologists' practices. If histochemistry is done on each core another $1800 is added.[74] In the case of academic medical centers, that money flows into the "teaching" hospital coffers. Even salaried urologists in prepaid HMO settings like Kaiser-Permanente are forced to do more biopsies than they think are necessary by lawsuits claiming delayed detection of cancer for lack of a biopsy.

One such lawsuit claimed loss of a chance at "cure" when PSAs of 237ug/ml and 239 ug/ml were not followed by a recommendation for a repeat biopsy after an initial negative biopsy.[75] A jury brought in a verdict of one million dollars for the patient even though, as the reader will learn in later chapters, such a prostate cancer must have been metastasing to the bone marrow fourteen years before those two initial high readings. Such verdicts force the medical-industrial complex to buy more PSA testing kits.

Muted criticism of the epidemic of testing emanates from the Master of Public Health brigade,[76] one academic urologist,[77] and one from the Mayo Clinic. The Mayo man found the "…overall yield from prostate biopsies has changed little during the last 15 years. Increased yield for men 70 years or older has been offset by the decreased yield in younger men."[78] The public remains unsophisticated in this matter[79] despite my letter published in the Wall Street Journal (WSJ) dated 5/9/00.[80] I have not been silent about this scandal.

One letter in WSJ by an M.D. does not change the course of civilization particularly when PSA tests (in these cases the % free tests quoted above) make a lot of money for Hybritech/Beckman Coulter, an automated instrument maker. They reported increasing sales from $1.2 billion to $1.9 billion from 1997 to 2001. The earnings per share and the stock price doubled in that time despite the "dot.com" crash. Of course, free PSA is a tiny part of their vast operation. My point is that medical testing is very profitable. Testing equipment is 67% of their business. Hybritech, a San Diego company which made the reagents for PSA, was purchased by Ely Lilly, presumably because it was profitable. Lilly continued to be profitable in the economic downturn of 1999 through 2002. Net sales increased 6% from 2000 to 2001. In 2003, Medicare paid out an estimated $38 million for PSA testing ($25.70/test) in men over age 75 in one year.[81] Individual practitioners can make profits doing it in their offices.

Nevertheless by 2003, disgust with the test among urologists had reached such a high level that Urology, what we call "the gold journal" and one of two major United States journals for the specialty, sponsored a print symposium on whether one needed to obtain a specific written consent to obtain a PSA. Members of the University of Chicago faculty were in favor of obtaining consent on several grounds: (1) the rejection of the screening concept for adenocarcinoma, cancers of glandular origin; e.g. the Danes rejected mammographic screening on the basis that the only two trials that reported death from all causes not just breast cancer showed no improvement; (2) screening for neuroblastoma in infants showed no improvement in the death rate and a 60% unnecessary surgery rate (3) and diminished insurability.[82] A Chicago internist felt that the idea of consent for PSA screening was poor because he thought unnecessary surgery in the elderly would be rare.[83] This internist was wrong. My inspection of a San Joaquin Valley (CA) hospital data base revealed 40 radical prostatectomies in men over 80 in the '85-'97 period. One just occurred in the twenty first century in a ninety year old, the father of a woman who works in my office. The internist quoted 29% over diagnosis rate in whites and 44% over diagnosis rate in blacks[84] but thought no ill would come of it.

A Massachusetts outcomes researcher concluded that PSA testing was no better than a lottery, my position in this chapter.[85] He cited the fact that the Seattle area with a prostatectomy rate five times higher than Connecticut in 1989 had the same death rate from prostate cancer in 2002. A Canadian has estimated that 94% of cancers detected by screening would not result in death from cancer before age 85.[86] A Georgia oncologist[87] quoted a 40% clinical insignificance rate citing the Canadians above and an Italian reference.[88] He also cited the well known failure of chest film screening for lung cancer, as well as the neuroblastoma screening study cited above. A Baltimore urologist cited (with approval) the M.D/patient conversation prior to PSA testing as required by the American Urological Association, the American Cancer Society, the American College of Physicians and the American Society of Internal Medicine.[89] My version of this conversation appears at the end of this book in the chapter called "Prescription."

A chairman of Urology in a Texas University organization balked at the idea of a written consent for PSA if other specialists are not required to obtain consent for their major interventions.[90] A Missouri professor of Urology cited a 60% false positive rate but went on to ignore his own critique and recommend screening without consent. The references he cited were "white papers" of the American Cancer Society and the American Urological Association, neither of which support his no consent position. Both currently require a "risks and advantages" conversation. Two Dutch urologists cited the Canadian McGregor study, the Italian Zappa study and their own which found 6 out of 7 screening cancers to be clinically insignificant.[91] They pointed out a study showing that the more that test patients knew about PSA screening, the less interested they were in undergoing it.[92]

Despite virulent criticism, screening with PSA continues.[93] PSA has become a "cashcow" for ambulance chasing lawyers. By "googling" "PSA-malpractice" I quickly found three cases which describe the ambience in which urologists practice today. (1) A PSA of 5.82 ug/dl was not followed up for four years. By then it was 41, and a bone scan showed numerous metastases, and there were enlarged lymph nodes in the abdomen. The case was settled two days before trial.[94] The problem with the settlement is that, as the reader has learned in this chapter, a reading of 5.8ng/ml has no specificity for cancer if 58 cc's of BPH/prostatitis is present. A reading of only 41 ng/ml when the lymph nodes were enlarged by cancer makes me think that this was an anaplastic cancer that made very little PSA because its DNA was so deranged. Such cancers present as a slight extra firmness without distinct borders within the BPH. Only the hands of senior urologists with extra experience in prostate cancer can reliably discriminate this from BPH with extra scarring from prostatitis. (2) A PSA of 4.1 was not followed up until two years later at which it was 4.8. Then it dropped to 4.5 in 12 months. Five years after the original elevation, the PSA was 10.2 and additional tests revealed "advanced cancer." The patient then was "injured" by a radical prostatectomy which was not indicated in my view. This case was settled for $400,000[95] although the initial PSAs were in the non-specific range. The PSA of 10 that lead to the diagnosis of advanced disease was just barely in Thomas Stamey's range for slight correlation with cancer volume. (3) A resident physician and his residency program were sued because he followed the American Urological Association recommendation that the M.D. discuss the pros and cons of PSA testing with a patient prior to drawing the blood. This person declined to be screened after the counseling session. A second physician at a later date ordered a PSA this time without seeking the patient's consent. It turned out to be very high and the patient was diagnosed with "advanced, incurable prostate cancer." A jury made a judgment against the residency program, not the resident, for a million dollars for sophisticated teaching.[96] They said in essence that physicians must give up excellence and act average to avoid liability; the physician's only obligation is to community standards, not published science. U.S. courts, in fact, have no settled policy about the separate existence of science as a body of knowledge that might be useful in deciding cases.

B. Konety of San Francisco found failure to diagnose prostate cancer was used to prove negligence in at least seven malpractice actions filed against physicians from 2002 to 2007 according to LexisNexis. "All of these actions have been settled or ruled in favor of the plaintiff. A previous study revealed that 29 lawsuits of failure to diagnose prostate cancer had been filed by 14 plaintiffs and settled for a total of $7.5 million. Of these lawsuits, 11 were determined to have been avoidable."[97]

But it is no surprise that these cases are not based on science. There are many analogous lawsuits against radiologists for supposedly missing small breast cancers via mammography and for missing small lung cancers on a chest film when they were supposed to be "curable." In regard to the famously successful "Pap" test for cervical cancer, 10 million women who lack a cervix (due to its prior removal with the diseased uterus) continue to have annual 'Pap' tests.[98] Cancer of the vagina itself is vanishingly rare. These "Paps" represent hysteria among our citizens and lack of probity by physicians who stand to make easy money from the worried well. None of the lawsuits that drive the madness, many successful for the plaintiffs, are based on science. Cancers that can metastasize do so at 2 millimeters in diameter, way below the specificity of any blood test, or computerized tomography (C.T.) scan. Much as I grieve with all M.D.s who have been assaulted by the legal system, I must say that the medical-industrial complex has brought these missed cancer suits upon itself by misleading the public in regard to (1) the trade offs between sensitivity and specificity characteristic of cancer screening tests[99] and 2) by the false promise that surgery/radiation can remove the cancer cells of the primary site of the common killers 'before they spread'. Gilbert Welch, M.D. of the Dartmouth medical school in Hanover, N.H., has trashed screening for most solid, interior, intrinsically metastatic cancers from a public health point of view at book length.[100] He excepted cervical cancer.

CHAPTER 4

The transrectal ultrasound guided biopsy: this is progress?

"Battling cascading steam, my ancient neighbor would face his fogged mirror, cutthroat razor mowing down, up piratical blade making every stroke a page torn from a life story told the hard way, because "Someone, by God, has to keep the old skills alive."–Leonard Cochran101

B y the early 1980s, progress in chip design permitted the miniaturization of ultrasound, namely a probe that fit in the rectum. This allowed marketing of ultrasound to urologists. By 2002, 73% of private practice urologists in the Western Section of the American Urological Association had ultrasound in the office.[102] At $50,000 per machine and assuming a similar percentage in the general membership of the A.U.A. that means there have been about $219,000,000 in sales of ultrasound equipment to the members of the American Urological Association since about 1990. This was mostly for transrectal biopsy.

At first General Electric and others marketed amortization of the cost in the office via an unstated but implicit claim that the image of cancer could be distinguished from normal, aged, prostate with its scars and calculi and benign prostatic hypertrophy (BPH). This implicit claim was disproved repeatedly. Eventually the American Urological Association stated in a white paper that "ultrasonography is not a useful test for early prostate cancer detection."[103] Cancers big enough to create a specific image can equally well be identified with the digital rectal examination.[104] This finding was reiterated in 2004.[105]

Moreover, this high tech transrectal method, new in 1983, did not find more cancers than the older technique. A study from Texas of the new technique in 1992 showed no significant advantage to the transrectal ultrasound technique over the transperineal technique.[106] Only four new cancers were found with the new transrectal ultrasound in 44 patients that were not found using the older technique. The fatal blow to the prevalent transrectal ultrasound technique, in my opinion, was a 2003 study in which the same patient was biopsied by both techniques; the older transperineal technique proved superior for prostate cancer detection.[107, 108] These results were confirmed by E. David Crawford of the University of Colorado in 2005[109] as follows: The perineal route "detected significantly more carcinomas than the (transrectal) route in both autopsy and prostatectomy specimens." In addition, the new transrectal route necessitated putting the biopsy needle in feces and then sticking it into the sterile solid prostate. That created an injury you might find on a farm! I stuck with the older transperineal technique both out of conviction and perforce, since the Veterans Administration was not going to buy a probe for a surgery service they were about to close in Walla Walla, Washington. From the citations above, you can see that it was no accident that eight out of ten biopsies I submitted there were positive for cancer. The ratio was reversed in the local private sector which was using the ultrasound- transrectal route to be modern.

Why, then, was the technically inferior transrectal ultrasound controlled biopsy technique with its inferior sensitivity adopted worldwide? There were four reasons. (1) It meant sales for equipment manufacturers, particularly General Electric. (2) The transrectal probe was physically easier for urologists, particularly as they aged; it's a long trip because of the obesity epidemic with the older, transperineal technique from the skin in front of the anus all the way to the prostate; trainees liked it because it was easy to learn. (3) Transrectal ultrasound provided a competitive advantage in a specialty with a twenty percent oversupply in manpower. (4) It paid more under Medicare. Competition within urology was fierce in the 1980s. When I was in private practice in Manhattan in the 1970s there were 250 urologists listed for New York City, a preposterous number. One hundred and fifty would have been plenty. Even today, I overheard a young urologist say that one of his hospitals in the L.A. basin (2.5 hours away from my former office in the southern San Joaquin valley) listed 67 urologists. The transrectal biopsy under ultrasound control looked then and looks now like "science" to the public.

The American Urological Association executive committee took the "high road" in their policy statement. They stated that the proper use of ultrasound was to facilitate thorough sampling of large volume prostates. The reader has learned in the chapter on BPH why sampling had become a problem: (1) benign prostatic hypertrophy (BPH), not cancer, was raising PSAs to levels above 4 ug/ml, the arbitrarily chosen action value. It was the new appearance on the clinical scene of these vast volumes which posed the sampling problem. In the pre-PSA days, we did not biopsy BPH, unless we felt the stony hard nodule characteristic of cancer with the rectal finger; (2) because the finger was no longer in the rectum to guide the biopsy needle, it became necessary to biopsy everywhere. Profits sky-rocketed.

As part of this vast, authorless deception that, like Topsy, "just growed," the benign prostatic hypertrophy (BPH) detailed in chapter 3 lost its name and became the "transition zone." This word concealed the fact that the "elevated" prostate specific antigen (PSA) levels which caused the biopsies were caused by benign prostatic hypertrophy,

BPH, not cancer. This neologism is an example of Orwellian propaganda, as discussed in later chapters on medical schools and intellectual life.

By 2000, the high false-negative rate[110] of the new technique was causing consternation within the specialty. To overcome poor performance of biopsies directed by PSA alone, urologists were urged to make ever more biopsies, first eight,[111] then twelve, then in 2004 twenty-one.[112] This last figure converts the prostate into Wendy's hamburger and has created ever higher pathology charges, up to $15,000,[113] since each core must be processed separately. Fee-for-service pathologists did not object to the increase in revenue, but salaried pathologists in the Veterans Administration system in Fresno groaned. Despite the frenzy, the cancer yield never improved over the percentage predicted by age as seen in Figure 1 of the chapter on BPH. The false positive rate for stand-alone PSA continues through 2018 stubbornly high at about 70%.

Transrectal ultrasound introduced a new problem not documented until fifteen years into the epidemic of care, a 15% to 30% false-**negative** rate. One study had a 30% positive biopsy rate the second time around in patients who had been negative the first time.[114] This same study featured nineteen patients with palpable nodules! These would have been positives the first time using the older finger in the rectum technique that I use. Instead, a 2003 publication suggested that the ultrasound probe be used like a giant finger to test the consistency of these nodules; the hard ones, they said, are cancer.[115] This was a bizarre suggestion. Why not just stick your finger in the rectum as I do, guide the needle into the hard spot, pull back to see that the nodule moves with your needle and pull the trigger? Why make a simple problem complex? I have been doing this for 40 years.

Another reason for the large number of false negatives, beyond the loss of the guidance of the examiner's finger, is the fact that via the transrectal technique the needle enters the prostate at a right angle. See Figure 1.

The transrectal needle samples very little of the compressed rim of true prostate, where the killer cancer lie, before it enters the benign prostatic hypertrophy (BPH) nodules that seldom harbor significant cancer. By contrast the older technique, coming up from the bottom, the perineum, what we call the apex, yields a long, oblique core of the rim of true prostate, where the killer cancers grow, often compressed by the presence of BPH centrally. This technique has recently been proved to yield more cancer in a prospective, but not randomized, trial against the transrectal technique. The perineal technique found 6% more cancers.[116] This was statistically significant. A 10% better cancer detection rate was found for the perineal route in a study of radical prostatectomy specimens.[117] I was one of the 3% of United States urologists who clung to the advantages of this technique. There are many more "old believers" in Italy[118] and Japan.[119]

Transrectal biopsy may have serious complications. Men have nearly exsanguinated after this procedure because of the proximity of the hemorrhoidal artery and the hemorrhoids, which are large veins.[120,121] For example, a sixty-nine-year-old otherwise healthy male presented in Montreal, Quebec, in urinary retention with a PSA of 75.[122]

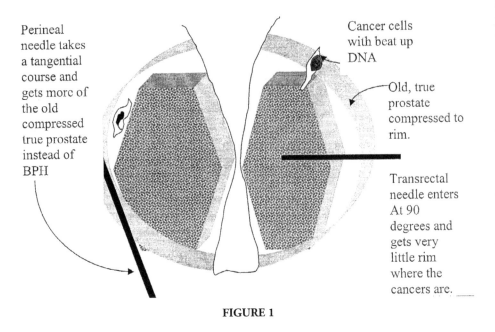

Perineal needle takes a tangential course and gets more of the old compressed true prostate instead of BPH

Cancer cells with beat up DNA

Old, true prostate compressed to rim.

Transrectal needle enters At 90 degrees and gets very little rim where the cancers are.

FIGURE 1

The perineal route finds more cancers because its tangential course samples more of the compressed true prostate. It is older than the BPH and contains, therefore, more errors in the DNA.

He presented ten hours after multiple transrectal biopsies with accelerating rectal bleeding and a low blood pressure. He was found to be consuming his clotting factors so fast that he could no longer clot the multiple punctures in his rectum. The artery leading to his prostate and penis on one side was embolized by radiology. He suffered acute renal failure, pulmonary edema, and bad rhythm in his heart. He left after three weeks. All the biopsies were positive for the highest grade of cancer suggesting that the ultrasound control was not necessary; one perineal biopsy anywhere in the prostate would have made the diagnosis along with a good feel of the prostate with a gloved finger. The authors suggest that patients with advanced prostate cancer, when bleeding from the rectum, should be investigated for a clotting disorder. I say that urologists should not cause ferocious bleeding in the first place; they should use the safer perineal route to stay sterile and dodge the big blood vessels.

Even worse are the infections to be expected when the biopsy needle is contaminated by feces prior to insertion into the patient's prostate. In one of the few head-to-head comparisons of the two techniques, 100% of the patients who had transrectal biopsy had bacteria in their blood (bacteremia) .[123] Twenty seven percent were symptomatic. By contrast, the transperineal route led to only a forty percent incidence of bacteremia; none of these cases were symptomatic. The organisms causing bacteremia via the transperineal route were skin organisms of lesser virulence. There is, to be fair, one report of an infection with the gas gangrene organism following the perineal route[124] but no deaths. This was probably caused by unintended entrance into the rectum because just below the prostate the rectum comes very close to the urethra. I have done that myself. In such cases, I treat the patient as though he already had septicemia.

Bacteremia is present in 16% of people subjected to transrectal biopsy who have not been pretreated with antibiotics.[125] On the other hand, pretreatment with antibiotics has not eliminated these dangerous infections. There was, for example, a 25% major complication rate in patients pretreated with tobramycin, a strong antibiotic.[126] Two percent of these patients required admission to the hospital. Others have reported a 28-37%,[127] 70%[128] and a 73%[129] bacteremia rate with a 44% incidence of shaking chills.[130] Sixty nine percent of patients not receiving a povidene-iodine enema developed bacteremia. This special enema reduced bacteremia to 19%, still high. Three of twenty five had positive blood cultures after a neomycin erythromycin base oral pre-op bowel preparation.[131] Stockholm, Sweden, reported a 3% hospitalization rate.[132] Others reported a 2% hospitalization rate without preoperative ciprofloxacin and zero with.[133] One of 625 patients needed to be admitted to the hospital in one series.[134] Brooke Army center reported that 4 of 670 (0.6%) needed hospitalization. If a single pre-operative dose of levofloxacin is given, the risk of symptomatic infection may be reduced to .25%.[135] Pre-operative enemas lower the incidence of this complication[136] but do not prevent it absolutely.[137] The very fact that there are so many studies of the issue tell us that there is an under-reported problem with the transrectal route. Under-reporting is equal to "publication bias." See the glossary at the end.

The Mayo Clinic reported in 1980, during the early days of this technique, seven patients who had undergone transrectal biopsy and who required admission for bacteremia .[138] The uncircumcised state has significantly more bacteremia (P=.003) than the circumcised,[139] an odd fact which may relate to social class, insurance status, and compliance with the pre-operative antibiotics protocol. The infectious complication rate was reduced from about 6.5% to 1.4% with pre-operative flouroquinones.[140] But flouroquinone resistant organisms have been described in patients undergoing transrectal ultrasound guided prostate biopsy in 1999[141] and 2003.[142] I consulted on such a patient in the intensive care unit with septic shock (hypotension) in 2008. He had been biopsied in another hospital. This is one way complications come to be under reported.

Then, there are the complications of septicemia, "bugs in the blood." For example, they have settled on the heart valves (bacterial endocarditis) in a non-diabetic despite ciprofloxacin given two hours previously.[143] A client of the Fresno V.A. hospital was referred to a tertiary hospital in San Francisco 3.5 hours away when they had the equipment for the transrectal biopsy under ultrasound and Fresno did not. For his 3.5 hours delay, the asymptomatic citizen began to grow bacteria on his heart valve, despite 'standard of care' pre-operative antibiotic. He required open-heart surgery to resect his infected artificial valve and re-implant a new one.

Here is a list of bacterial complications of transrectal ultrasound obtained from a PubMed search, in chronological order: 1979: **death** from E. coli sepsis;[144] 1978: 2

patients with anaerobic septicemia;[145] 1982: E. coli meningitis;[146] 1983: E. coli bacteremia and non- Clostridial crepitant cellulites;[147] 1984: polymicrobial septicaemia due to Clostridium difficile and Bacteroides fragilis;[148] 1992: Osteitis pubis;[149] 1992: Acute pyelonephritis;[150] 1993: **death**; anaerobic infection following transrectal biopsy of a rare prostatic tumor;[151] 1997: Adductor myonecrosis;[152] 1999: **death** from Clostridium sordellii ischio-rectal abscess with septicemia;[153] 1999: **death** because of a multi-resistant strain of enterobacteriaceae;[154] October 2002: **death** due to septic shock;[155] December 2002: an infected disc space;[156] August 2004: septic shock. Total deaths = 5.

Due to publication bias complications are under-reported. For example, in a 2003 report from an academic venue on this topic, the authors claimed to have found no reports in the literature of septic shock or death.[157] They could not have looked very hard because, I found the **five deaths** above quickly in a routine internet search of the National Library of Medicine at a free site called Pubmed.

Transrectal biopsy causes a small but measurable mortality widely scattered over time and space. In contrast to the Challenger disaster, visible to the whole world, these deaths are collated here for the first time. When reported as a percentage of the millions of prostate biopsies, these deaths have flown beneath the "radar screen" of my specialty. When aggregated to absolute numbers, as I will do for the mortality of radical prostatectomy, the problem is more serious. Assume a .007% death rate,[158] a biopsy rate of 1890/100,000,[159] and a conservative conversion factor of five. These assumptions yield an average of **66 deaths per year** in the five year period 1993-97 just after the peak of the epidemic. Using that figure, I estimate the number of deaths from transrectal biopsy in the period 1984-1997 to have been, in the Medicare population, **nine hundred and twenty four**. In about six hundred, the biopsy probably was negative for cancer[160] and these are deaths of healthy citizens who do not yet possess a serious diagnosis! I heard of a death in the private sector of Fresno when I suggested to a veteran that I biopsy his prostate. He looked at me as though I had suggested he go before a firing squad. He said that his neighbor had just died of infectious complications of a prostate biopsy. This death was not published and therefore, according to the current fashion of evidence based medicine did not occur. I reassured the veteran that my technique was different from that which killed his neighbor. I mentioned these deaths to David Crawford, Prof. Urol. and U. Colorado, after he gave us a lecture at the Western Section of the A.U.A in 2008 about the ins and outs of cancer negative PSA directed biopsies. He said he had never heard of a septic death of this sort. At the same lecture session Michael Brawlely, M.D., of Seattle, who has spent a professional lifetime wrestling with the poor specificity of PSA, disclaimed knowledge of a septic death following transrectal biopsy. I am not surprised at these denials. They both work in big city referral centers. These complications tend to go to different hospitals than the hospital that caused them. For example, in the fall of 2008, I was called to the intensive care unit of my hospital to attend a man in septic shock caused by a transrectal biopsy in a smaller hospital 20 miles away.

If we use data from a non-Medicare source, my figure of 924 dead is an overestimate. For example, in a county whose data is dominated by the younger, wealthier, privately insured patients of the Mayo clinic, the peak utilization of prostate biopsies was only one quarter of the Medicare peak.[161] It averaged 288/100,000 during the epidemic, about one sixth the Medicare rate. If we use a less conservative conversion factor, 10.38, from the 1992 census for the population over age fifty in the whole country, this would yield **251 dead** nationwide from the contaminated, transrectal technique in a twelve-year period 1980-1992. Five deaths have been published in the literature. This gives a ratio of one published death for each actual thirty-five deaths in my estimate, a measure of publication bias. I heard of three more published deaths at the Western Section of the A.U.A. at Vancouver B.C. meeting in August, 2011. But there is no journal of bad results. Associate professors of urology do not get tenure by writing such papers.

The total cost to the taxpayer of prostate biopsies using $119, an average between the in and out patient Olmstead County Medicare rate, comes to $4,268,920 for the 12 year period, $711 per urologist (assuming 6,000 active). This leaves out the facility hospital fee and the cost of the complications which are much larger.

CHAPTER 5

A history of radical prostatectomy to the present day

"Who would have thought the old man had so much blood in him?"
— Lady Macbeth

As surgical technique improved in the late nineteenth century on skin cancers that only killed by local extension, not metastasis, surgeons were tempted to apply it to interior, intrinsically metastatic cancers. The failure of lumpectomy to lengthen life quickly became apparent in the case of breast cancer. William Halstead of the newly founded Johns Hopkins Hospital hypothesized from the failure of lumpectomies that a wider excision would improve the cure rate which was zero. He started, as an experiment, to take the breast with its skin, the underlying pectoralis major and minor, and the regional lymph nodes in the arm pit. Neither he, nor anybody else did a randomized control series of lumpectomies. There was no control series of lumpectomies in man or animal for the next 65 years. His nineteenth century operation, still an experiment, was still being done at Columbia Presbyterian Hospital in New York eighty years later when I trained there in the early 1970s.

I did four of these operations as a general surgeon in the Air Force. The muscle excision made the arm useless; the lymph node dissection caused chronic lymphedema of the arm. Lymph nodes are not dispensable. Claudius Galen said, "Everything has a purpose." Lymph nodes do. I recall solving a persistent accumulation of plasma under a skin flap caused by the interruption of the lymphatics using a combination of aspirin and antihistamine,[162] a trick I learned during my student research days. I did these operations under the supervision of a fully trained general surgeon from the Ann Arbor Michigan program, Bruce Robinson, M.D. I hated the operation at that time and I suspect he did too. But a surgical residency is one long obedience exercise. Surgery arose from the military, not the university. I was a captain in the Air Force and was not about to start a revolution.

Hugh Young's radical prostatectomy for cancer arose directly from William Halstead's experimental procedure on women. Halstead assisted at the first radical prostatectomy in 1905.[163] The provenance of the operation was Albarran's nineteenth century publication of a 14% incidence of prostate carcinoma within the nodules of benign prostatic hypertrophy (BPH). BPH was beginning to be shelled-out of the rim of compressed true prostate. The incidence of cancer in benign, smooth muscle tumors (BPH) has not changed significantly in 100 years. Albarran's observation was rediscovered in 1989.[164] Young thought in 1910 that, as in a tuberculous abscess, early excision would give better results than late.[165] Unfortunately, "early" is not early enough. Contemporary tumor biologists tell us the average diameter at which metastases begin may be as early as 250 micro millimeters, or .25 mm.[166] This is one tenth of the two millimeters in diameter routinely cited by students of the metastatic process[167, 168] as the time when metastases begin. Oncologists in private practice carry a 5 millimeters diameter in their heads[169] but 2 millimeters is a "basso continuo" of this book. The Halstead/Young uncontrolled experiments in humans that never passed before a review board were confounded by the fundamental biology of metastases from the very beginning.

In contrast to the radical mastectomy, the medical community did not "buy in" to Young's radical prostatectomy for many years. From his first report, we can see why. The first patient was totally incontinent during the day. Six months later Young wrote, "… he began to suffer pain in the urethra. Examination shows three calculi in the bladder. Operation, lithalopaxy (*crushing the stone with forceps*). One calculus was found attached to a silk ligature and in removing this, the mucous membrane was torn. This was followed by a perineal abscess, extravasation of urine and death four weeks later…autopsy showed…behind bladder along left vas deferens was a small area of carcinoma."

My comment: Young reported the condition of the patient as "excellent" for six postoperative months despite the notation of gross, total urinary incontinence and the finding of residual cancer at autopsy. This is French deconstruction. The meaning of Young's adjective "excellent" is fluid. In Hugh Young's lexicon it can mean the opposite! The second patient died seven weeks postoperatively of "infection in both kidneys." The third had urgency incontinence six months later and had cancer at the margins. The fourth patient was totally incontinent and was lymph node positive for cancer. Young stated, "There was no operative mortality." True, there were no deaths within thirty days of the operation. But at its heart, his statement is not true to the plain meaning "operative mortality." Both cases one and two should be called operative mortalities. Their deaths were only delayed six months and seven weeks post-operatively. Death from wound infection is typically delayed. For Young to say there were no "operative mortalities" was a public relations gimmick typical of surgeons looking to generate more income from referrals.

Such deaths from bacterial infection were characteristic of the old days. He cheerfully concluded, "The four cases in which radical operation was done demonstrated its simplicity, effectiveness and the remarkably satisfactory functional results furnished."

An editorial comment in the Journal of Urology on the reprinted article dated February of 2002 agreed by stating, "Dr. Young… identified a safe surgical procedure."[170] This statement is not true; the procedure was not safe for the three out of four men who died of infection after 30 days, nor for those with obvious residual cancer.

In regard to the safety and efficacy of the procedure, not everybody in the first half of the twentieth century missed the fact that two of the four patients died of complications. Despite modifications in the postwar period *e.g.* Robert Lich's adoption of the English retropubic approach over Dr. Young's approach in front of the anus, and despite the advent of blood banking and penicillin, by the early 1970s the operation had left the repertoire of academic urologists. For example, the chief of Urology at Memorial Sloan Kettering in New York told Cornelius Ryan, author of *The Longest Day*, that he was trending away from the operation. In 1973, the year I finished my urology training, the Journal of Urology contained no articles about radical prostatectomy.

The operation had been abandoned because academics knew that the semblance of cure was explained by the prolonged natural history of the disease. Robert Lich, Jr., M.D., a chairman and professor of Urology at Louisville, Kentucky, gave up the operation after two patients with apparently complete resections died of metastatic disease 27 and 28 years after his radical surgery.[171] The prolonged natural history was quantified in 1995. It was determined to be 52 years. The doubling time is 475 days. Hugh Young had recognized the prolonged natural history in 1905. He wrote, "Cancer of the prostate remains for a long time within the confines of the lobes and especially the posterior capsule of the prostate resting inviolate for a considerable period of time."[172] He also recognized that "the involvement of the pelvic glands (lymph nodes) occurs late and often the disease metastasizes into the osseous (bones) system without first invading the glands."

A 1974 paper defined Dr. Young's "considerable period of time." It said, "There were no cancer deaths for the 68 patients (6.5%) in the lowest prognostic categories 4 to 6. For the 302 patients (29%) in categories 4 to 8, the cancer death rate was so low that a serious question arises as to whether they should be subjected to any potentially dangerous treatment unless (and until) signs or symptoms develop which indicate that they are actually suffering progression of their cancer. The data for stages III and IV patients with histologically low grade cancers suggests that these patients are at no greater risk of death from cancer than most stages I and II patients for whom radical prostatectomy has been recommended (and was performed in this study)."[173]

This government-sponsored understanding of the natural history of the disease governed attitudes toward the operation in the 1960s and 1970s. It led to the frequently cited randomized, controlled, prospective Veterans Administration study of radical prostatectomy, May 1967-March 1975. This was much discussed as oral history during my urology residency. It was aborted by a denial of funding by congress in 1978, a penny-wise/pound-foolish decision. The first formal publication of the results appeared in 1981.[174] I remember a furious debate ensued within the specialty in which a proponent of radical surgery pointed out that there was a "66% chance of overlooking a 50%

improvement in survival and a 50% chance of overlooking a 66% improvement."[175] This was true due to low enrollment. The Veterans Administration finally found it necessary to restart a randomized study of the operation 28 years later. Accrual has been completed and, at 750 men accrued to the experimental radical surgery side and 750 to the control unoperated side, it is way short of its announced goal of 2,000. As of ten year results reported in 2011, there was no significant difference between radical prostatectomy and surveillance only even though the radical side, because it was margin positive 30% of the time, tended to get androgen ablation early. It, like the Swedish study, is confounded by the tendency of the radical surgery side to get early androgen ablation before the control side.

The second line of evidence that led to the almost complete abandonment of the operation by 1973 was the evidence first reported in 1934, that even the earliest, incidental, occult prostate cancers discovered at autopsy had metastasized to the perilymphatic spaces of the nerve supply of the organ.[176] This observation haunts the apologists for radical excision to this day.[177] The cancer deposits signify metastases have occurred, and not only to perineural lymphatics. Even Hugh Young, in 1910, recognized that the cancer's best soil was the bone marrow. It multiplies there and kills by acting as a metabolic sink rather than by local extension, as in the case of cancer of the cervix.

When I was a urology resident in the 1969-73 period at the Columbia Presbyterian Hospital in New York, it was commonplace for us to aspirate the bone marrow for prostatic acid phosphatase. This recognized the primacy of the bone marrow as the home of choice for wandering prostate cancer cells. The bone marrow aspiration needle put a pit in the center of our hands because of the force necessary to push it through the cortex of posterior superior iliac spine. If the level of the enzyme in the bone marrow was higher than the serum level, we presumed metastatic disease and cancelled any planned radical excision. A private practitioner in the far West told me that in the 1990s he used to aspirate the bone marrow for prostatic acid phosphatase but that he got so many high readings that he could not make a living. He stopped aspirating the bone marrow as B.F. Skinner would predict.

Today, there are two new techniques for detecting metastases to the bone marrow, (1) polymerase chain reactions, PCR, and (2) monoclonal antibodies, selective immune proteins. The second, the monoclonal antibody technique, is more reproducible. For example, epithelial cells were reported to have been detected in the bone marrow of 54% of patients undergoing radical prostatectomy.[178] That is proof that the radical procedure cannot cure. The data above were reported at 7:25 a.m. October 25th, 2002, in a research forum far from the plenary session where routine clinical matters were being discussed. I was there with, perhaps, five people in addition to the presenters and three moderators. The results were later published in Urology, the second most important journal of urology in the United States. The early hour, the separation of the two venues, the slightly less prestigious peer reviewed journal, illustrate how the medical industrial complex protects itself against data that might lower cash receipts, with publication bias.

The rates of detection via PCR are higher, 90%-75%, but it is much harder to replicate. O.J. Simpson escaped the consequences of his presumed actions because PCR is so tricky. Even though similar data has been presented by laboratories on three continents for a variety of cancers including prostate,[179, 180, 181,182] this line of evidence is usually dismissed by apologists for the radical as not ready for prime time. Another typical criticism of the data is to say that these bone marrow aspirates have never been correlated with clinical deterioration. This is not true. They have been on multiple occasions.[183] For much more on this, see the chapter on bone marrow aspiration. Even though basic clinical science was against it, the rate of radical prostatectomies began to accelerate in 1984 after years of decline. The percentage of patients treated dropped slowly from 8% in 1974 to 7% in 1983. The rate then accelerated in 1987 when prostate specific antigen (PSA) testing was introduced. This was the beginning of the catastrophe for men and women. The percentage of patients treated with surgery tripled from 1984-1993.[184] The rate per 100,000 quintupled. See Figure 1.

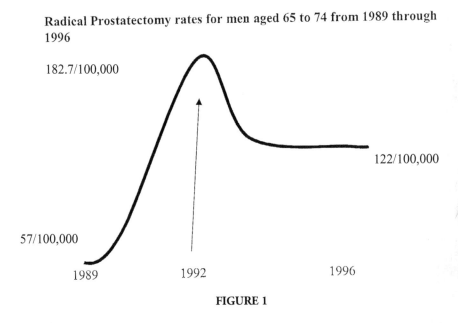

Radical Prostatectomy rates for men aged 65 to 74 from 1989 through 1996

182.7/100,000

122/100,000

57/100,000

1989   1992   1996

FIGURE 1

Rates abruptly declined when Medicare said it was going to study the utilization of radical surgery in those over 75, an age they thought inappropriate. [185]

The reason radical surgery regained favor was a report by P. Walsh, M.D., in 1982 from John Hopkins, Hugh Young's bully pulpit of 1905, that suggested that erectile potency could be preserved despite the operation.[186] Dr. Young did not mention sexual function in his paper, a sign of his puritanical times. The 1982 paper held that, "it is incumbent upon urologists to perfect surgical techniques so that fears about the morbidity of the procedure do not discourage patients and physicians from selecting the optimal form of treatment." There was no data to support the notion that radical surgery was optimal in 1982. There had only been the VACURG study with insufficient numbers to draw any conclusion. Moreover, I do not recall myself or my fellow young attendings in the 1970s being in a mood to deny our patients a cure of cancer because of our unwillingness to cause impotence/incontinence as a complication. Instead, we spoke of the cancer as being intrinsically metastatic at the time of presentation and of its high incidence at autopsies when it was not the cause of death. I recall an attending urologist just starting at Columbia Presbyterian Hospital in New York viewing, with disgust, a film showing widespread bony metastases a mere six months after he had done a radical prostatectomy for cure. He said he would never do another. He said the operation was nonsense and advised me not to do it. This operation peaked in utilization in 1992 and then abruptly declined. The cause, in my opinion, was "a new approach to quality assurance in Medicare" published in the Journal of the American Medical Association.[187]

This was code for, "We are going to kick you out of the Medicare program if you keep doing radical prostatectomies in persons over the age of 75." Those who carried out the initiative deny their decision to collect data had any effect except in Arizona.[188] They point out that the actual statewide information programs began in 1993-95, but the numbers fell off a cliff a year earlier in 1992. By contrast, I believe that the mere announcement of the intentions to crack down in 1992 was sufficient to terrify the urologists whose hands were inappropriately lodged in the federal cookie jar. The Peer Review Organization actions appeared to have an equal effect on control hospitals, which received no extra information about the Sheikh and Bullock study, as much as on target hospitals. The controls were contaminated, in my opinion by the fact that urology is a small specialty. Urologists are full-time gossips. Word of mouth spreads quickly. Many urologists knew by 1992 that they were being watched, that they were skating on thin ice.

Radical prostatectomy rates decreased 75% from 1992 to 1997.[189]

In Olmstead county, home of the Mayo Clinic, the rates were cut in half from a peak in 1990 to a trough in 1994. Outside the Medicare age group the absolute number of those having the operation while under the age of sixty increased fivefold between 1989 and 1995; under age 55 the rate increased eightfold.[190] These increases proceeded in the absence of data which showed that cancer specific life was being prolonged in animals or man. The first randomized and prospective series that purported to show cancer specific life extension in man was published in 2002.[191] The public should not fall on their knees and worship this paper. The lives saved did not drop to the bottom line to show up as an improvement in death-all-causes as they should have. In a follow-up paper they claimed cancer specific life extension of 5%. But the series was confounded beyond redemption by the fact that the radical surgery group had the benefit of early androgen ablation while the watchful-waiting group did not. This paper will be extensively analyzed in the chapter on the role of the universities.

The epidemic of treatment with intention to cure rages on. A national hospital based figure reported at the American Urological Association (AUA) meeting in April 2018 in San Francisco, which combined both high and low utilization areas, showed a 9.01% decrease for standard open radical prostatectomy rates while robot-assisted radical prostatectomy declined 8.6%, 2012-2014. Both rates have been unchanged for 2014-2015. This contrasts with another national study by nine high volume referral centers with longer follow-up which showed a 22.6% decline in surgical volume of high risk cancers in 2012-2016 compared to 2008-2012.

Fewer biopsies are being done in the United States. In July of 2018 James T. Kearns, MD, clinical fellow of urologic oncology at the University of Washington School of Medicine (327 radicals/100,000, a utilization only exceeded by Alaska; see figure 1, chapter 6) reported that the rate of biopsy per 100 patients who underwent PSA testing fell from 1.95 in 2009 to 1.52 in 2014 as a result of the USPTF ruling. Of those who had a new cancer diagnosis, the proportion who received definitive therapy (meaning radical surgery or radiation for putative cure) fell 15% (HemOncm Today, July 25th 2018, page 44). Definitive therapy for prostate cancer is not a growth business in one of the highest utilization states and university-based medical schools. All U.S. medical schools are going to have to find a new source of income since all have participated in the epidemic.

My personal stance on eliminating the primary site has been nerve sparing cryosurgery using the third generation equipment purveyed by Endocare. Using liquid argon for the freeze portion, helium for the warming portion, and transrectal ultrasound to monitor the advancing edge of the ice ball, I have been able to spare the nerves to the sphincter and to the penile vessels. The destruction of the primary site has a theoretical advantage of 1.5 years of life gained. This is inside the standard deviation of the mean time to death from PSA discovered cancers, i.e. 1.7 years. Any life gained could easily be due to chance alone. With proof of benefit statistically impossible, focal elimination of the primary cancer must have no physiologic losses to preserve the principle of beneficence i.e. no provable gains must be matched by no losses. My patients seem to be reassured that something, cryosurgery, has been done about the primary site and happy to have their erections and urinary continence. The return of immunotherapy of cancer to public consciousness in 2018 makes cryosurgery even more acceptable.

CHAPTER 6

Geographic variations in rates of radical prostatectomy and radiation

T he coincidence of the 1992 peaks and immediate steep declines of the rates of radiation and radical surgery rates in the United States, Canada, and France[192] suggest that broad cultural forces in the developed world are at work to aggravate an epidemic sparked by the introduction of PSA and transrectal ultrasound. There is no chance that the pool of citizens with significant prostate cancer could have been depleted at precisely the same time all over the developed world.

But what kind of anthropologic data leads us to the answer? The study of extreme geographic variations provides a hint. For example, in Fresno California, the radical prostatectomy rate per 100,000 (Medicare-non-HMO) was five times the Manhattan rate in 1992.[193] This extreme difference persisted through 1995. Fresno, like New York, had grand opera and free summer Shakespeare in the park, but its aggregate of wealth, brains, and artistry is quite different. Fresno does not represent the smart money compared to New York City. Rates across hospital referral regions may vary 7.8 times across hospital referral regions.[194]

Similarly drastic geographic variations have been found in knee arthroplasty,[195] lower extremity revascularization, carotid endarteretomy, back surgery, and colonoscopy. Such operations show two-fold (arthroplasty) to ten-fold (back surgery) variations across hospital referral regions.[196] In the case of colonoscopy, large numbers of procedures were found to be associated with decreasing appropriateness.[197] By contrast, there is no such variation for hip pinning for fracture of the hip, a diagnosis about which there can be no argument.

Robust inferences about the cause of drastic geographic variations are almost absent from the medical literature.[198, 199] The authors express puzzlement at the vast differences in the rates of mostly surgical procedures. But they are not surgeons. I am one and feel free, therefore, to present my own case study and draw conclusions.

Consider the differences in utilization rates of radical prostatectomy between the Northeast United States and the West. The western states, where rates are high, are big and thinly populated. If states with high-utilization are depicted according to their land area, it looks as though most of the United States bought into the high rate of radical surgery mentality. But if a map of the United States is redrawn to be proportionate to Electoral College votes,[200] radical prostatectomy wins only 60% of electoral college votes. Fully 40% of the country dissented. See Figure 1.

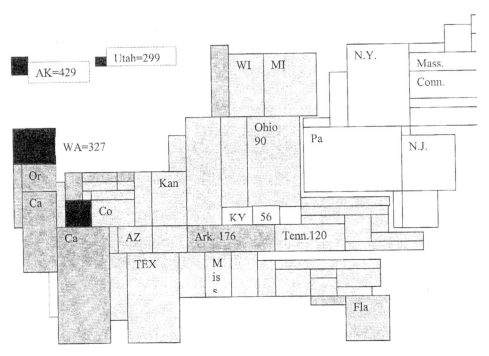

FIGURE 1

Frequencies of radical prostatectomy/100,000 in the United States with areas proportionate to Electoral College strength. The white areas represent radical prostatectomy rates of <75/100,000 Medicare beneficiaries 1988-1990. Grey=75-149, dark grey=150-224, black=>225. Note that the Kentucky rate of 56 is half its neighbors.

The Northeast and Kentucky dissented from the epidemic.[201] That is a lot of folks. Areas south and west of the Mason-Dixon Line, except for Kentucky, dove into the maelstrom. The Alaskan rate per hundred thousand was twenty-one times the Rhode Island rate; the state of Washington rate was six times the Kentucky rate. Why? One published clue is a difference in attitudes toward radical prostatectomy for advanced age groups between the Northeast and the rest of the country.[202] The Northeast did fewer radical prostatectomies as the patients passed age 75. In the Pacific and Mountain states, the opposite was true. The eighty-five-year-old father of one of the women in my California office had a radical prostatectomy in 2007. This was unwise. He did not live 30 days. As citizens passed age 75 in Utah, they had more radical prostatectomies. This Utah effect becomes even more drastic in the greater than age 80 group. Seattle had a similar enthusiasm for operating on the elderly.[203]

It is important to note that, even in a state such as Wisconsin with one-third the rate of Utah and Washington, the rate for radical prostatectomy more than quintupled from 1984 to 1990.[204] This prompted howls from the Wisconsin Department of Health and Social Services. They were paying under Medicaid. They wrote, "surgical treatment has not been shown to be more effective than other therapies."[205]

Let us turn the question around. How do we explain the low-rate states, *e.g.* Kentucky? To research that anomaly, I contacted the former chairman of urology at the University in Louisville, Mohammad Amin, M.D. According to him, the Kentucky story was as follows: the previous chairman of urology, Robert Lich M.D., had eagerly embraced the radical prostatectomy in its post-World War II English retropubic form. At the end of his thirty-year career, however, he was appalled to see two of his earliest cures come into his office with metastatic prostate cancer at 27 and 28 years. He advised his successor to the chair of urology, Dr. Amin, to eschew the operation. Dr. Amin did just that at the cost of personal income. Nor was Dr. Amin's Lich-inspired stand popular with the Urology Residency Review Committee. They criticized his low rates of radical surgery. Ultimately he left the university to join the V.A. where he felt no pressure to do radical surgery that he thought was unwise. The science-based position of these two academics set the tone for the entire state of Kentucky in 1992. Its radical prostatectomy rate was half that of its neighbors. When I called Dr. Amin to ask him about his state's low rate, he could not understand how I had spotted Kentucky. I said his state stood out like a lighthouse in a storm at night.

Utilization rates of radiation for putative cure have drastic geographic variation similar to that of radical prostatectomy. For example, Connecticut had a rate one quarter that of Seattle.[206] But there is a caveat here; Connecticut substituted radiation for radical surgery in the seventy to seventy-four age groups. Connecticut is an outlier in that respect. Their radiation rate is 20% greater than that of Utah, the outlier on the high side in radical prostatectomies in the lower 48. And so, Connecticut has nothing much to crow about as a bastion of scientific care.

The party line on these variations has been to refer vaguely physician uncertainty about the science.[207] This is an evasion of the uncomfortable issue of social class in the United States. It is the patient population, not the physicians, that varies with location.[208] The published correlations with radical surgery rates are sociologic namely, age >75, in the West,[209] marriage,[210] and the presence of insurance. Absent any more cogent published correlations by medical sociologists, I have found others in the annual statistical abstract of the United States[211] and in the Dartmouth Atlas of Medical Care.

I wondered if attitudes toward surgery in general varied from the Northeast, defined as New England plus New York, Pennsylvania and New Jersey, to the far West, defined as the states beyond the Rockies plus Wyoming.

The results showed that the Western United States is more enthusiastic about surgery of all kinds compared to the Northeast defined above. There were, for example, 7% more radical mastectomies than lumpectomies in the West. Shoulder surgery increased dramatically in the traverse from East to West.[212] There was an identical 75% increase in back surgery for slipped disc and radical prostatectomy rates moving from the Northeast to the West. Disc disease is a condition of high prevalence with advancing age and uncertain significance just like prostate cancer. The TURP rate fell a statistically significant 9% moving from Northeast to West in 1992. Radical prostatectomy was substituted for transurethral prostatectomy (TURP) for benign prostatic hypertrophy (BPH) in several areas.

Indices of social disorder coincide with the West's rapturous attachment to surgery. Teenage pregnancy, as a percentage of all pregnancies, increases from 9 to 12% percent (P=.005) moving Northeast to West. It is a plague among the white Anglo-Saxon Protestants in Wyoming where I worked for four years. Income decreases significantly (P=.01) from 24,000 to 21,000 dollars per year Northeast to West. Suicide is 70% greater and auto accidents double, Northeast to West. I calculated significantly **positive** Pearson correlations between radical prostatectomy and teenage pregnancy, auto accidents, suicide, and back surgery. See Figure 2.

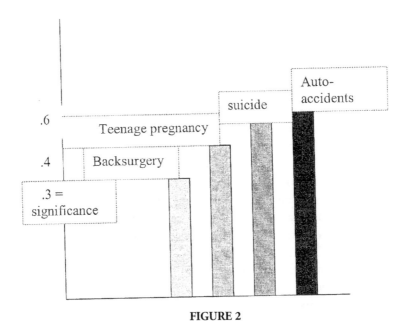

FIGURE 2

Pierson correlation coefficients between radical prostatectomy and three social indices plus back surgery. Above .3 is significant. Auto accident is the strongest correlation.

I found significant **negative** correlation between the TURP rate for BPH and income. A detailed look at the correlations by state between income and percentage radical prostatectomy done for all cancers discovered appears in Figure 3.

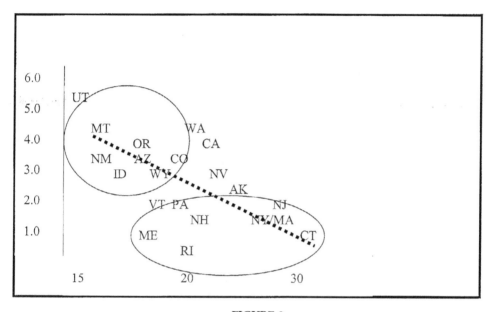

FIGURE 3

Percent radical prostatectomy per 100,000 (vertical axis) versus income in thousands (horizontal axis) in Northeastern states compared to Western states. Higher income correlates with a lower percentage of radical surgery.

Correlation is not causation. That mantra said, this data is consistent with the hypothesis that it is patients' cultures and social class that varies with geography more than the doctors' ideaology. It is true that different cultures attract different types of doctors. Geography alone explains less than 2% of the total variation in the use of radical prostatectomy.[213] Geography is often a reflection of social class. Social class is verboten in the U.S. This data says that the best marker for who will get a radical prostatectomy is not where they live but who they are. Let's face it. The people I took care of in Wyoming, oil and gas roustabouts, were Sam Sheppard's people, solid enough to have a good, hazardous job with health insurance. They were of northwest European extraction, usually England and Ireland. The divorce rate in Wyoming is 70%. Some have been, like myself, rock climbers. They do not delay gratification like yuppies of the Northeast. More than two years of college is not common. They want action.

It is not only the males who are Sam Sheppard characters. The female populations, moving East to West, make similar choices about surgery related to similar social indices. For example, in New Mexico, we know that 57% of instances of intraductal carcinoma in situ, not cancer in the layperson's sense, are treated with total mastectomy versus only 28% in Connecticut.[214] Social predictors of total mastectomy are a lack of a college degree and lower income levels.[215] Eight years after the peak of the epidemic of surgery, no improvement in prostate cancer specific survival was found in areas with high radical prostatectomy rates.[216,217] The 8 to 11 years follow-up in these studies is not enough time to see a difference. But the fact that geographic studies are published at all signifies disbelief among the cognoscenti that the epidemic of radical prostatectomy and radiation will/can improve the death rate per hundred thousand.

Geographic differences in patterns of care in prostate cancer of similar magnitude exist internationally. The percent of newly diagnosed patients considered candidates for radical surgery may differ two-fold between European university hospitals.[218] Seventy-nine percent of respondent American urologists would choose radical prostatectomy for themselves for an apparently localized tumor whereas only 4% of British urologists would.[219] In 1999, only 25% of United States urologists used the prostate specific antigen **density** to filter out the false positives caused by BPH/prostatitis, while in Canada, 37% did.[220] American urologists are twice as likely as Canadians to involve medical oncology with early, asymptomatic hormone refractory disease.[221] Within France, prostate cancer mortality can vary two-fold between provinces.[222] Clearly science is not the sole paradigm determining utilization.

Lynn Payer, formerly a reporter for the New York Times, related such differences to the method of insurance payment elected by the country in question. Her father subsidized her book during the two years of its writing.[223] No publisher would pay upfront for this kind of news. For example, she reported that Belgian surgeons are paid for the repair of lacerations by the number of sutures. Their work looks like the repair of a rent in a balloon. English surgeons are paid by the length of the incision. They find far fewer sutures to be adequate. She correlated the exact type of medical insurance chosen by her four study countries, England, the United States, Germany, and France with the underlying culture. She died young of breast cancer with all medical policy wonks in her debt. Her book is often in the syllabus of medical policy courses in our major universities.

CHAPTER 7

Two complications of the radical prostatectomy: death and urinary incontinence.

"When beggars die there are no comets seen. The heavens themselves blaze forth the death of princes."–Claudia in Shakespeare's Julius Caesar

The epidemic of radical prostatectomies and radiotherapy, indeed this book, would be of no interest if the two modalities had only trivial biologic complications. The price would only be money. But the apologists for both modalities pitch their procedures as though there is no biologic price. This is important to them because, to make the medical-ethical claim of beneficence, a favorable ratio of good to bad, the complications, the denominator, must be said to be zero because the numerator, life extension, equals zero. Life extension has not been demonstrated for either radical surgery or radiation in a properly randomized, controlled, prospective series. When the numbers are aggregated as I do here, rather than presented as percentages, the cardiovascular deaths within thirty days, erectile dysfunction, and urinary incontinence add up to a huge penalty for United States citizens, male and female.

Here is a description of a death within hours of a radical prostatectomy that occurred in California. "We are standing beside my husband's body, in a small private room on the surgery floor... I am crossing myself compulsively, out of some archaic, nearly forgotten impulse from my Catholic childhood whispering fragments of the Our Father and the Hail Mary to myself...Cold. He is warm but getting colder. I kiss his mouth, his beard, his beautiful grey curls... My daughters and their friend are sobbing, gasping, even cursing next to me."[224] This is how Sandra M. Gilbert, a published poet and professor of English at U.C. Davis, described the death of her husband, Elliot, the chairman and professor of English, in 1991. He was a man so charming that his daughters as toddlers pleaded to ride with him when he went to the grocery store. To balance this one death, there has to be a whole lot of good to come out of radical surgery but there is not.

He was part of the epidemic of surgery in younger men I graphed in the previous chapter that, in 1992, replaced the epidemic in those greater than age 75. His death, because he was only sixty and privately insured, went unrecorded by the Medicare Administration. Medicare is by far the best source of metrics regarding the epidemic because it is national and non-selective in its data. By crosschecking with the Social Security Administration death notices, they have a good idea of what is going on. Medicare has published that the thirty-day mortality for radical prostatectomy in 1991 in the age group covered by the program was 1%.[225] This sounds small but it quadruples the expected thirty-day mortality for the age group. Peri-operative mortalities of 1% do not customarily excite the attention of surgeons when the surgery has been shown to prolong life e.g. appendicitis or gall bladder surgery. Andy Warhol died after a gallbladder operation. Gallbladder surgery did not cease nationwide to await the outcome of an enquiry such as that concerning the Challenger disaster. The reason there was no outcry is that gallstones can kill you. If gallbladder stones get loose in your common duct, and if bacteria get there too, you can easily die. Also, gallbladder surgery is curative in the usual layperson sense of the word. In the case of prostate cancer, surgery has not been shown to be curative and it does not cause death within the actuarial life span of most people who harbor it.

But the word "cancer" has been coupled with these postoperative deaths. It throws up a protective fog around the 1% statistic. For more impact, I have estimated the absolute number of deaths in the Medicare age group, 1984 to 1998, using published surgery rates[226], the 1% mortality Medicare figure, and the data for those over age sixty-five from the 1990 census.[227]

One percent is conservative for the 30-day mortality because it was more than twice as large, 2.45%, in 1988 in Canada.[228] I cut in half the resultant absolute number for each year up to 1993 because the estimated numbers of radical surgeries by population turn out to be twice the actual Medicare insurance claims for money.[229] After 1993, I have used actual numbers of claims, not estimates, for radical prostatectomy.[230]

With these procedures, the number of deaths within thirty days of a radical prostatectomy in the fifteen year period was **3,753**. Of course, this elderly group of patients is not guaranteed against death within 30 days even if they had stayed home. Because the Medicare administration estimated, as noted above, that the operation quadrupled the baseline death rate for the age group, I subtracted 25% of the total from the total. This gives **two thousand eight hundred and fifteen** excess deaths for the period 1984-'98. This is an underestimate because almost 2% died in the greater than 75 age group; 4.5% died in the older than eighty-year-old group.[231] The father of a woman working in my office in Delano was one such. These elderly caused an upward bump in prostate cancer mortality after the introduction of PSA testing which peaked in 1992. See Figure 1.

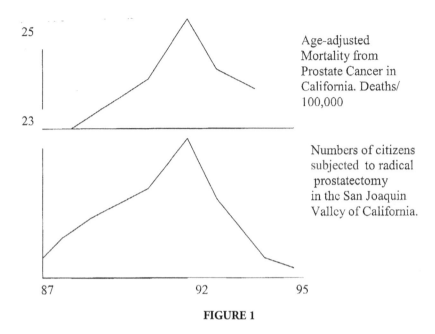

FIGURE 1

The Pearson correlation coefficient between the all California death rate from prostate cancer and rate of radical prostatectomy was **.7** in the years 1987-95 when PSA screening became common place.[232,233] .3 is considered statistically significant. There is no escaping the conclusion that this spike in deaths represents post-op deaths from radical surgery.

The total cost to the taxpayer for urologists' services for the period using the 2000 Medicare payment of $1849 for radical prostatectomy was $1,044,614,738. Private practice charges averaged $6,370, a fantasy figure, an opening gambit. Hospital charges for the period were, using $16,990 per operation[234] or $9,598,704,380.00. N.B. On average nation-wide hospitals collect 47% of charges. That makes total collections for hospital and urologist $1,064,331,912.00.

This is big business. The 2,000+ excess deaths drew no attention from the media because they were scattered over time and space. They have never been totaled before the writing of this book. They are visible as a peak in the 1992 graph of the annual United States prostate cancer mortality statistics. There was an increase from 22 to 25 per 100,000, the California number, in 1992, the peak radical prostatectomy year. The death rate then dropped to 23 per 100,000 the following year.[235]

These huge changes in a statistic that changes little from year to year have been missed by medical journalists. It is a matter of the scale of graph design. The death rate is usually presented on the same scale as the prevalence rate of cancer. Since there is only one death for every 380 cancers present in the population, the upward deflection looks like Mt. Everest from the moon. It seems like a little blip of no consequence.

Even data from upscale areas and university practice plans show a near doubling of the death rate from 1987 to 1992,[236] the peak year for radical prostatectomy. Their death rate dropped to baseline in 1995 after radical prostatectomy rates had declined by 40%. The increase of the prostate cancer death rate for blacks with the advent of PSA testing was even more dramatic. Their death rate jumped from 51 to 55 per 100,000 between 1987 and 1989, the years of introduction of prostate specific antigen (PSA) screening,[237] a fact duly noted by Patrick Walsh, the chairman of Urology at Johns Hopkins.[238] The black death rate peaked in 1993. For whites, the increase in the death rate began gradually in 1983 at less than half the black level, peaked in 1991, and ended at 25 per 100,000 in 1995. A similar peak of deaths occurred in 1992 in Quebec at 33 per 100,000, a huge figure.[239] These prevalence figures have had no impact on the medical press because absolute numbers are left out of the picture. Few know the result of dividing 100,000 into various populations. They cannot therefore do the aggregate numbers in their head, and so the epidemic of post-operative death has gone unrecorded by the press.

At least one group published concern. Public health experts have written in a peer reviewed forum that the rise in the published death rates was caused by "…a statistically significant probability of overdiagnosis of prostate cancer death when the underlying cause of death determined from information in the hospital records was compared with that of the ICD-9 coding rules… *This situation occurred most frequently when…a patient died after surgery.*"[240] They could not bring themselves to say that the men died of clots in their lungs and/or coronary arteries within 30 days of operation. Major surgery increases the viscosity of blood. Twenty-five percent of persons with significant coronary artery disease have no symptoms particularly if they have no habits of exercise. This, plus under-transfusion of packed cells, as I read between the lines, is why Professor Elliot Gilbert died.

Since the mean time to death for the stage of prostate cancer typically discovered by PSA testing is seventeen and a half years,[241] the abrupt decline in the death rate after 1992 cannot be due to a lifesaving property of the operation. All stakeholders are willing to stipulate that. Salaried government scholars have ascribed 60% of the improved thirty day mortality to a decline in the frequency of the operation in the elderly (poor risk) category.[242] Some say death certificates are accurate.[243] I do not. There is a bias in the private sector toward not reporting postoperative complications. Few residents in training will write, sign, and date that the operation done by the chairman, who will write their letter of recommendation for their next position, killed the patient with his surgery and not the cancer.

As a case study of this hypothesis, consider Professor Gilbert's death certificate. In a university hospital, these are filled out by interns and residents, M.D.s dependent on their superiors for a salary. The first cause was said to be cardiopulmonary arrest, a tautology. It says he died because he died. The second cause listed was liver failure. Nonsense. The liver does not fail in four hours. The third cause listed was prostate cancer. I believe that, when this certificate arrived in Sacramento to be tabulated in the annual cancer statistics, his death was misattributed to prostate cancer instead of hypoxic injury to the myocardium as a result of major blood loss. No M.D. charged with the job of entering him in the books in Sacramento would find number one or number two credible. Who says an M.D. does this job? It could be a sophomore in college with a summer job from political influence. Number three is not accurate either, but it has a flicker of rationality sufficient to tempt a non-specialist late for his tee time. And so we see a notable jump in prostate cancer deaths in 1992 via an orgy of amateurism.

Who cares about **2,615 excess deaths** except their widows? Apparently, the Medicare administration noticed because they funded a study of time trends, geographic variation, and outcomes of radical prostatectomy published in 1993, a year after the peak of the epidemic.[244] The geographic variation was found, in turn, to relate to differing attitudes toward the aging of the patient. In the West, the older you were, the more likely you were to have radical surgery. In the East, the older got less radical surgery.

The Commission for Disease Control (CDC) in Atlanta smelled a rat. They sponsored an International Conference on Prostate Cancer Screening, Early Detection and Control September 6-7, 1995, three years after the peak of the epidemic. Several final statements were drafted by conference chairs,[245] which included the statement, "The patient should know all his options (including expectant management) prior to treatment." The reporting in the American Urological Association's Health Policy Brief went on to say, "There is no conclusive data on the long-term efficacy of current treatments…The conferees could not agree on a blanket statement regarding the best treatment…researchers must look at data *beyond ten years* for definitive answers regarding treatment…It is hoped that the CDC's published summaries of the meeting will interest practicing physicians, State and Federal Health Officials.…" Amen from me!

The promised summary was never published. I telephoned the CDC in 1996 to ask, "Why?" A civil servant speaking slowly and guardedly told me that there had been so much strife over the drafts that no publication was possible. The lack of consensus in 1996 caused the CDC to hold a second convocation on the same topic five years later, in December 2000. This time the recommendation on the CDC website was for an informed consent before drawing a PSA, as though it were a surgical procedure. The CDC is now funding a study of communication between black men and primary care physicians about cancer preventive messages.[246] To me, this is an implicit statement that informed consent is not possible on such a subtle issue. A book is necessary, in my opinion the book you are reading, to inform fully.

The Medical Board of California became involved. They issued a policy statement in 1994 called "Treatment of Prostate Cancer." It said that a notice about prostate cancer treatment options must be available to patients. During the breast cancer wars they had required the same list of options regarding radical mastectomy. In essence, it was a republication of the January 1994 information provided by the National Cancer Institute of the United States Public Health Service. It did not inform the public that the word "options" is a term of art in health policy circles, the same error made by the American Urological Association in its pamphlet.

If any urologists missed the brouhaha in the mid-nineties, there was a flurry of lawsuits to alert them. Professor Eliot Gilbert's wife, Susan Gilbert, settled and sealed her suit for the wrongful death of her husband. Not everybody settled. For example, on December 1st, 1991, six days after a radical prostatectomy, patient D.B. jumped out of a third floor window to his death and caused a judgment against the nurse in charge.[247] A death caused by an extensive myocardial infarction after radical prostatectomy was settled for $350,000.[248] A fatal pulmonary embolism following wound dehiscence was settled for $175,000.[249] There was a suit claiming that the urologist should have told the patient about the more conservative alternatives available which had equal claim on his attention.[250] A veteran named Thomas D. Murray, age 65, bled to death one day after a radical prostatectomy at the Veterans Administration hospital in north Chicago. His widow claimed 3.5 million dollars in punitive damages.[251] Claims related to "prostatectomy" were the most expensive in a survey of urologists' malpractice cases from the St. Paul Company from 1995 to 1999.[252] St. Paul Company has since left the malpractice business. All these must have been part of the suddenly diminished enthusiasm for Dr. Walsh's revived prostatectomy after 1992. It is not whether a suit is won or lost that determines a doctor's insurability. It is the fact that the suit is brought at all.

The second major complication of radical prostatectomy and radiation is loss of sexual function for the male and, secondarily, the female. To this, I devote a separate chapter which follows.

The third major complication of radical prostatectomy is urinary incontinence. Again absolute numbers portray what I have seen as a practicing urologist better than the sterile percentage figure. The three year postoperative Medicare data show improvement from 20% in 1991 (the peak of the epidemic) to 4% in 1995.[253] Nonetheless, 4% of a large number is a large number. Quite a few of them began to show up in my clinic at the Walla Walla Veterans Administration hospital starting about 1987. In this case, let us multiply the number of deaths above, estimated at 1%, by four to get **11,260 cases of incontinence**, a substantial underestimate because the rate was 20% in 1991.

Urinary incontinence is degrading to the male psyche, focused as it is both on control of others and self control. A 1996 Canadian study showed that 8% of men who were incontinent of urine after radical prostatectomy were suicidal.[254] If applied to the United States total, it means we would have, in addition to the deaths within thirty days, **450 men with suicidal ideation**. A 2004 Finnish study found a 3% incidence of *actual suicide* during the deliberations of a panel on the cause of death in prostate cancer screening.[255]

Artificial sphincters in this older age group are fraught with infections and erosions and so one cannot say that there is a nifty solution to post radical prostatectomy incontinence. By contrast, stress urinary incontinence in the female is less of an assault on female self-esteem, in my experience. Incontinence with coughing or laughing is often caused by the happy event of childbirth. Some women have what we urologists call giggle incontinence even when teenagers. Funny movies are not a bad association for incontinence. By contrast, for men, the condition represents a drastic loss of status, competence, seniority.

Why is there incontinence in the post 1983 nerve sparing era? The reason is that prior to the operation quotidian urinary continence does not depend on the outermost, red, voluntary muscle fibers wrapped around the urethra at the outlet of the pelvis. It depends instead on white, involuntary, smooth muscle at the bladder neck. This is where minute-to-minute continence resides at every age group. The outer, red, voluntary sphincter only comes into play when coughing, laughing, or lifting. I have cut right through the outer red muscle sphincter in two patients with fractured pelves, hitched the urethra directly to the prostatic urethra via a transpubic approach exactly as is done in radical prostatectomy, and found that these young males were continent minute-to-minute after the operation. To be sure, they did have to hurry to the bathroom at the first sensation of fullness.

By contrast with an operation tailored for traumatic disruption of the urethra, radical prostatectomy must, perforce, interrupt the white, involuntary, smooth muscle of the internal sphincter at the bladder neck. If it does not, it is a sham radical because it does not take adjacent tissues uninvolved in the cancer as a precaution against local recurrence. All that remains after a true radical is the voluntary, red, striated muscle of the external sphincter. This muscle has been shown to be subject to programmed cell death[256] as part of the aging process. These cells can renew themselves just so many times and then they die, one of the reasons the truly elderly have trouble hanging on to their urine even without an operation. Implantation of a multicomponent artificial urinary sphincter is not a realistic solution since there is a 5% to 10% risk of infection and 25% to 50% percent need for surgical revision.[257] Where is the beneficence of that? Thus, the graduates of the 1992 epidemic of care who live thirty years will surely have vastly more incontinence than their unoperated age mates. There are no studies funded and ongoing of controls and operated patients to refute this hypothesis.

Let me sum up the costs of the epidemic. For one billion dollars, the United States suffered a public health catastrophe from 1984 to 1998 consisting of an estimated 2,815 thirty day postoperative deaths, 118,642 impotent, less happy (worth $59 million per year) men, 118,642 sexually frustrated, less happy (worth another $59 million) women, and 11,260 incontinent men (450 of them suicidal). This occurred without the proof of life extension in man or animal that would satisfy the committee on medical experimentation at Neuremburg.

CHAPTER 8

Sex after radiation or radical surgery.

SINNERS WELCOME
"I opened up my shirt to show this man the flaming heart he lit in me, and I
was scooped up like a lamb and carried to the dim warm. I who should have
been kneeling was knelt to by one whose face should be emblazoned on
every coin and diadem:

No bare-chested boy, but Ulysses, with arms thick with hard-hauled ropes.
He'd sailed past the clay gods And the singing girls who might have made
of him a swine. That the world could arrive at me with him in it, after so
much longing- impossible. He enters me and joy sprouts from us as from a
split seed."[258] —Mary Karr, Atlantic Monthly, Oct. 2004. p. 129.

N ow that is the voice of a woman who enjoys sex. Our urology literature, and
general interest books by senior women, give hearty endorsement to the idea
that women over 50, 60 and 70 with (even without) steady partners enjoy and value
sexual intercourse in its classic form. Kimberly Ford, a Ph.D. in Spanish and French literature from Berkeley, has written that woman in the reproductive age do not feel tip-
top unless they are having 2-3 orgasms a week.[259] The bad news about radical
prostatectomy and radiation[260] is that the impairment of sexual function by radical
surgery and radiation has been under-reported, an example of publication bias. For
example, despite the advent of detailed studies of female sexual arousal by urologists[261,262] there has been only one publication detailing the female response to the
post-radical prostatectomy penis.[263] It was a questionnaire study. Only 52% of male
patients returned the questionnaire at one year. Publication bias is the tendency of all
peer reviewed journals to publish only results that increase revenue to the faculty practice plan. To correct this bias, I called all the non-responders to mailed questionnaires
failures. That said, only 20 of the original 91 (22%) of patients' partners gave the Viagra inspired "partial erections" a score of 78%, *i.e.* total satisfaction. Viagra commonly
inspires headaches[264] because it dilates arteries everywhere not just the penis.

One objective metric for the post-prostatectomy losses suffered by women is the loss of one to two centimeters in length in 19% of one prospective series.[265] Twenty-three percent of women report that length and girth are important in sexual stimulation.[266] Women describe increasing orgasmic intensity with increasing depth of massage of the vagina.[267] Patrick Walsh, M.D., former chairman at Johns Hopkins, claims that shortening does not occur when the procedure is properly done. He says the bladder is extensively mobilized downward during the operation to prevent shortening. This extensive bladder mobilization is not described in the literature at large. In fact, he describes the opposite "…if there is any tension when pulling down the bladder, a Babcock clamp is used to hold the reconstructed bladder neck in place while the sutures are tied."[268] Even if extensive mobilization of the bladder were done, the bladder will retreat. Its attachments to the pelvis will haul the penis back to its pre-op location. One of my patients at a V.A., a Yale graduate and more articulate than most of my vets, described the shortening of his post-radical prostatectomy penis with considerable bitterness.

Actually, penile length is an important stimulant toward orgasm in some women. Less than four inches was said to frustrate orgasm by one porn star.[269] But most testimony holds that width is more important.[270] Width is probably a surrogate word for hardness because, as width increases, the columnar shape of the erection is less deformable by lateral forces. Artistic foreplay is also critical. "A book of verse, a jug of wine, and thou beside me singing in the wilderness. This is paradise enow."[271]

The evolutionary purpose of penile erections is, in addition to sperm transport, clitoral massage to orgasm. Orgasm produces the peak partial pressure of oxygen in the plasma filtrate which is the vaginal lubricant. The spermatozoa need that much oxygen to swim through the cervix. There have been so few studies of the proper technique for clitoral massage that Kim Cattrell of the television show, "Sex in the City," wrote a book about it, *The Art of the Female Orgasm*. She could find no descriptions of exactly how a man might best induce orgasm in a woman. From the point of view of evolution, there has to be some kind of peak pleasure from intercourse for the female. I have seen on the Discovery Channel a very big African male elephant mount a small female. His size and tusks must have been alarming to her. To turn your back to such a creature would require positive reinforcement equal to the fear induced. Among humans in missionary position, resistance by the penis to lateral deformation is necessary to apply pressure to the clitoris when the ventral portion of the penis is pressing against the back wall of the vagina. The clitoris is supported by the pubic bone as a fulcrum. The engineering formula for bending stiffness is a constant (B) times the end force (the pressure of the ventral tip of the penis against the back wall of the vagina), times the initial force (pressure applied to the clitoris support by its fulcrum, the pubic bone) divided by **the cube** of the length. A long penis must be thick as well in order to apply sufficient pressure to the clitoris. Dorsal deformation of the penis against the pubic bone has been depicted with magnetic resonance imaging.[272] Most post-radical prostatectomy patients report a stuffable penis,[273] more balloon than bone. The initial force, *i.e.* pressure on the clitoris, must be diminished (1) by failure of the penis to fill to maximally and (2) shortening of the penis considered as a lever arm by two cm. There are no studies of what the pressure must be to lead to orgasm.

The urologic publications we have about post-radical prostatectomy sexual function are almost exclusively from the male point of view about vaginal penetration. Vaginal penetration records resistance to axial deformation *e.g.* a nail being pounded into wood. This predicts female satisfaction in the case of virgins only. Even in that case, penetration is only a beginning. Orgasm is not guaranteed. It is only the midpoint of what women wish to be a ritual lasting at least fifteen minutes[274] in this age group. Well-meant publications directed at the post-radical prostatectomy market which extol non-traditional methods of female satisfaction have to admit that "there are times when we both miss the old, no-fuss erections."[275]

In the twenty-first century, there is no doubt that sexual selection occurs by female choice. Certainly it explains the peacock's tail which would be a real drag on its fortunes in the forest otherwise. Among insects, in species where the females mate with many different males prior to conception, the penis has twice as much variety as those that mate with only one male.[276] This suggests an attempt by the male to set himself apart from his competitors. Among humans, "The Dyak men of Borneo use a palang, a smooth bar with rounded ends made of bone or metal, to transect the head of the phallus. Dyak women, according to anthropologists, say that sex without a palang is like unsalted rice, but with it, it tastes like rice spiced with salt."[277]

The few studies in the penile prosthesis literature of the female response to erections of varying quality point to a different experience than that reported by the male. One found that female partners subjected to inflatable prostheses were more content with the sexual experience than females subjected to malleable prostheses.[278] Male contentment was about the same. Another study found that after an implant of a third-generation inflatable prosthesis, 70% of the men judged their sexual activity as "excellent" while only 28% percent of their partners thought the prosthesis to be excellent.[279,280] This was more than a two-fold difference between male and female perception of penile quality.

A loss in a function so deeply conserved as reproduction cannot be dismissed as a small event even though in this case we are dealing with persons in their fifth, sixth and seventh decade. The achievement of these life spans is so recent that I do not believe our brains have adjusted. Surely evolution would cause female excitement to occur with bone hard, not stuffable erections. Stuffable would suggest to the female a genetic defect in the male that might lead to weak offspring.

Clitoral massage to orgasm, in addition to convincing the female that the exposure to big, rough males is worthwhile, has a function critical to the survival of the species; it provides the peak oxygen tensions in the vagina necessary to stimulate motility in the spermatozoa long stored in a low oxygen environment in the cauda epididymidis. The partial pressure of oxygen in the vagina before sexual excitation at 3.8 mm Hg is too low for spermatozoa to function. Sexual excitation creates arterial dilitation, venous constriction, genital swelling and a transudate of plasma into the vagina with a partial pressure of oxygen at 28 mm Hg, a sevenfold rise.[281] All that wetness is not a glandular secretion; it is oxygen-rich plasma squeezed out of the vascular tree by the blood pressure. While the thermal and vibratory thresholds for the clitoris and vagina have been published,[282] there is no data on what pressures on the clitoris by the penis are maximally excitatory at what time during intercourse. The solitary experiment I found in the literature designed to test pressure was terminated because the first and only subject found the excitation was too intense. In my private practice, a 50 + year old woman complained that the 30 degree deviation of her husband's penis toward the ceiling due to Peyronie's disease, a sort of arthritis of the penis, denied her the usual pleasure of intercourse. Although he was content with the quality of their intercourse, she was not. Again we have, as in the case of penile prosthesis above, a dichotomy of experience with the same organ.

There are those that tell us that "The lovin' ain't over."[283] Barbara and Ralph Alterowitz have written a fine book about sexual function after radical prostatectomy and irradiation. It actually supports my main point here. They emphasize that female sexual excitation is based more on touch than the male, which is more visual. It seems to me that a bone-hard erection sensed by touch must be far more exciting (because sexual selection is by female choice) than a stuffable erection caused by the two main interventions for so-called cure discussed here. I have no data to support that statement; it is an inference from my knowledge of general biology and years in the clinic. The "lovin" may not be over but it surely is not the same from the female point of view.

Women acquire the same amount of happiness from sex as men.[284] In fact, sex four times a week has a very large effect on happiness, particularly among the highly educated.[285] Two to three times is necessary for maximum happiness as quoted above. Changing a habit from once a month to four times a week creates the same amount of happiness as an extra $50,000 of income[286] so says the *Wall Street Journal*. In the light of that data, a couple in their low twenties that I interviewed prior to a vasectomy must have been rich indeed. He said their habit was three times a day. He fixed home appliances for a living, so I guess he returned to his house at noon.

She looked very relaxed despite two children running around the office. I have heard twice a day from a couple in their forties in Delano.

That an active sex life with a man may be important to the happiness of women over sixty can no longer be in doubt after the publication of the book by a retired Berkley High School teacher of English, Jane Juska.[287] When she retired, she decided that she had not had enough sex in her life, and that she would remedy the deficit by placing an ad in the New York Review of Books which read as follows, "Before I turn 67 next March, I would like to have a lot of sex with a man I like. If you want to talk first, Trollope works for me." She got 66 replies and explored four of them in detail. This is not an uncommon situation. A strong desire for intercourse by women in their sixties and beyond is as well documented.[288,289] The losses women suffer in this area highlight the lack of beneficence of radical prostatectomy and radiation. Relative to

61

post-radical prostatectomy patients across all time points, their women partners have reported lower general quality of life.[290] This might be because "Your first ejaculate will be urine"[291] as related by the 2008 president of the Western Section of the AUA about his own radical surgery. Or the lower quality of life might be because of a diffuse slackening of sexual activity. Sex and happiness are strongly correlated.

If both nerves are spared, the claim is that erectile function satisfactory to the male can return in about 70% of those who had good function preoperatively[292] *e.g.* Robert Dole. However, none of the published studies promoting radical surgery and radiation tell us what happens five years later. My education, training, and 35 years experience tell me that age related functional losses after the two modalities will be accelerated compared to unoperated, unirradiated controls.

Of particular concern in that regard, is the oft noted, but heretofore unexplained, loss of desire for intercourse in the post-radical prostatectomy male. He can "get it up" with the help of Viagra, vacuum suction devices, injection therapy directly into the penis, massage by his lover, but he does not want to. This is not a mystery. It is caused by the loss of a sense of fullness in the prostate which would, if it were present, send reflex afferent signals to the spinal cord. The cord returns efferent signals to the arteries of the penis that cause them to dilate, the veins to close, Meissener's corpuscle to become more ticklish, the bulbocavernosus muscles to spasm and the subsequent erection to become bone hard. A man wants to have intercourse when his prostate is full of semen. No semen. No desire. Much semen, much desire. Sex for men is not an intellectual event. There is little free will involved, as one of our recent presidents has stipulated. Buddhism preaches that the way to happiness is to stop desiring but my experience with both men and women after the loss of testosterone is that the loss of desire is experienced as disease.

If we calculate that, of the 70% of those who are potent pre-operatively, 30% become impotent post-operatively, we end up with **118,642 men with new impotence** in the epidemic years. To represent the females' loss of consortium, we should double that to **237, 284 persons with unsatisfying sex lives**. Kim Cattrell, of "Sex in the City" fame, tells us that, until she found "an artist" at female sexual stimulation, sex without orgasm was irritating rather than satisfying.[293] This artist became her husband. I think we should listen to her *vox clamantis in deserto*.

CHAPTER 9

Radiation for Prostate Cancer

"As early as 1902, the first case of X-ray induced cancer was reported... Early radiologists and dentists manifested a significant increase in skin malignancies and leukemias as compared to physicians who did not use radiation." —Syllabus on fluoroscopy radiation protection. California Department of Health Services, Radiologic Health Branch. 6th revision, p. v, p.65.

Between 1983 and 1996, 61% of patients with a new diagnosis of prostate cancer in a private practice setting had some form of radiation. Its administration correlated with insurance and income.[294] But, radiation given early obviously does not control metastatic deposits of carcinoma cells in the bone marrow any more than surgery does. See the next chapter on metastases. The situation is worse in regard to control of the primary site. The consistent failure of radiation to achieve even local control of this particular cancer has been common knowledge among attending urologists, urology residents, and even medical students since the 1930s. Radiation with cobalt failed before World War II. Modern iterations fail now because the beta ratio of irreparable to reparable damage to the DNA is very low at 1.5 as opposed to 10.0 in the radiosensitive tumors.[295] The reason is the prolonged doubling time. See the chapter on prostate cancer as an exponential function. DNA unraveled in preparation for mitosis is three times more susceptible to radiation than the DNA of interphase cells.[296] One almost never sees mitosis among middle grade prostate cancer cells, the most common type.[297] In fact the surrounding fibroblasts undergo mitosis more often, and therefore are more sensitive to radiation than the prostate cancer cells. This is the reason radiation sometimes burns a hole between the urethra and rectum.

Moreover radiation also up regulates clusterin,[298] a tissue messenger whose job it is to persuade cells not to commit the suicide ordinarily programmed into their DNA. Human prostate cancer cells that have been irradiated are up regulated toward immortality 84% by doses up to 30m Gy.[299] Gy is a measure of radiation intensity. The word radiotherapy is therefore, oxymoronic. It is not therapeutic for prostate cancer.

Since radioactive cobalt was tried in the 1930s, a succession of radiation sources have failed amid a slew of complications. Examples are radioactive gold at the University of Iowa, Iodine 131 or 124 seeds at Memorial Sloan Kettering, and supervoltage at Stanford in the 1970s when Cornelius Ryan was diagnosed and then seeds, this time palladium, again.[300] Seventy-eight percent of patients with locally extensive prostate cancer given supervoltage had positive biopsies two years or more post radiation.[301] This sublethal injury to the DNA causes the cancer to be more aggressive than it was to begin with.[302,303,304] Peter Carrol and Garry Grossfeld of U.C. San Francisco published in 1998 that the mitotic index was doubled by radiation and that the ominous P53 gene, a regulator of proliferation and cell suicide, occurred in 54% of irradiated cancers versus 8% of non-irradiated cancers.[305] I routinely biopsy irradiated prostates when the patients come in for voiding symptoms. I need to know whether it is predominantly BPH or residual cancer causing the symptoms. I see crazy looking residual cancer cells all the time. In my mean time to death series at the V.A. in Fresno published in the British Journal of Urology, all the vets who had been irradiated but not given immediate anti-androgen deprivation were dead within 10 years, which was an unusually quick exit for this series and statistically significant.

Because of its carcinogenic effect, radiation causes vast suffering. It triples the incidence of bladder cancer.[306] These cancers and rectal cancer[307] occur 5-10 years after the radiation and so usually escape publication as complications. I took care of a wildly anaplastic[308] aggressive bladder cancer in the V.A. in Fresno in a non-smoking high school teacher who had been irradiated for cancer of the prostate. The bladder cancer looked like something from science fiction under the microscope. His wife asked me, "Whose idea was that?" I tell you this. It was not mine.

As mentioned above, radiation can cause colonic ulcers and fistulae to both the perineal skin and the rectum. Michael Sarosody, M.D., reported four colostomies in 170 irradiated patients for these conditions in 2003.[309] Moreira et al reported 11 more at a 2003 section meeting. One of their patients died. If it does not cause a fistula it may still cause miserable burning and frequency of urination remediable only with hyperbaric oxygen. There were two such in Sarosody's series. Twenty percent of his series could not urinate at all for a median time of 55 days. One of my patients at the V.A. in Fresno lost his urethra completely. I went looking down a tube that ended in an obliterated pinhole. Talk about a low beta! I had to put in a permanent suprapubic tube. Like new cancer induction, these complications occur as long as thirteen years after the radiation.[310]

Because of its low beta, radiation injures arteries more than it injures prostate cancer cells. Only 55% of men retain erectile function two years after external beam radiation.[311] Radioactive seeds have an impotence rate 20% better than external beam at two years. This has been used as a marketing ploy by Theragenics, a seller of seeds.[312]

64

But two years is wholly inadequate to document the effect of radiation on arteries. Ten to fifteen years is more like it. This will be when we see the carcinogenicity of the 17% incidence of radioactive seed migration to the lungs.[313]

Seeds have become big business since Andy Grove, the chief of Intel, described how he chose them in a 1996 article in *Fortune* magazine.[314] His PSA was 5.0 ug/ml, in the non-specific range *vis a vis* prostatitis and BPH. A middle grade cancer was found on random biopsy. Unlike Robert Frost's narrator of "Two Roads in a Wood," he chose both roads, the systemic route of androgen ablation, and the local route of seeds. 120,000 seed implantations have been done in the last 15 years.[315] Seeds were 36% of treatments for seemingly localized prostate cancer in 1999. When seed implantations are added on top of the falling radical surgery rate in 1997, the total treatments with intent to cure almost equaled the height of the surgery epidemic.

The seeds as a cause of radiation-induced complications have been no better than external beam. Jorge Lockhart, M.D., *et al* of Florida reported in 2004 eighteen patients in the previous three years with "…devastating complications following brachytherapy in the treatment of prostate adenocarcinoma." There were eleven connections between the urinary tract and the colon plus seven bladder neck contractures. Two of them developed unusual radiation-induced cancers. One of these died as a complication of replacing his bladder with a new bladder made of his intestine.

The latest wrinkle on radiation is so called conformal therapy, meaning the external beam will be sculpted so that it hits only the prostate, not the rectum or bladder, in doses purported to be lethal to cancer. The problem with this pitch is that it is the same as that given for supervoltage in the 1970s, cobalt in the 1930s, and radioactive gold in the 1960s. A conspicuous 'silence' surrounds the demise of supervoltage as I write in 2019 with the exception of a paper by Christine Gray, M.D., *et al* of the U.S. Navy. They documented the continuance of prostate cancer specific deaths twenty years after radiation.[316] Worse, half of those left alive had signs of cancer necessitating androgen deprivation. Only 15% of those eligible for evaluation had no evidence of disease at 20 years. It is no surprise that the bad news came out of a socialized medicine scheme. My guess is that 0% will be free of evidence of prostate cancer at 30 years.

Radiation was pitched in New York to Cornelius Ryan in 1970 in tortured English as offering a "potential expectation of cure."[317] Ryan smelled a rat but bought anyway. It may have hastened his death by causing further injury to the DNA of the cancer. His cancer probably became more anaplastic and less obedient to neighboring fibroblast commands to cool it. Radiation was finally denounced in print within my specialty in a peer-reviewed publication by Thomas Stamey, professor and chairman of Urology at Stanford, where M. Bagshaw began the fashion for supervoltage years before, as follows: "I hope that most physicians will recognize that radiotherapy is no longer a viable option for the treatment of prostate cancer. We should not use a therapy that can make 80% of the patients worse than the natural history of the disease."[318] In 2004, Neoptolemos J.P. *et al* demonstrated the same aggravation of cancer specific death in regard to pancreatic cancer.[319]

It is hard for the medical industrial complex to admit that radiation to certain cancers is harmful because it makes so much money for the university medical centers and for the suppliers. For example, the income statements of Theragenics, the sole U.S. supplier of palladium seeds, showed an increase in gross sales from 25 million dollars in 1997 to 50 million dollars in 2001, a 100% increase.[320] These dollar sales have since declined due to "price pressure" in the U.S. market. This led to the sale of Theragenics Corporation to the privately held Juniper Corporation in 2013. Juniper then sold it to CR Bard Corporation where it resided briefly until purchased by Becton Dickinson in 2017 to create a worldwide behemoth capable of distributing the seeds throughout the world.

These declines in dollar amount of sales have not discouraged Christine Jacobs, the president and CEO of Theragenics. Gross profit was, after all, 65% of revenue in 2002. She sees growth in this market. In the 2002 annual report she pointed out that "six thousand baby boomers turn 50 years old every day…Additionally, more women…are voracious in identifying the treatment options for men. Nowadays, women, as well as men, will have a say in whether or not their men are impotent or incontinent."[321] She placed an ad in the Atlantic monthly in the July-August issue of 2003 which referred to "one happy significant other," an allusion to the typical joy of sex for women and that there is less impotence at two years caused by seeds as compared to radical surgery. She presumes Atlantic monthly readers are ignorant of the low beta ratio of prostate cancer in response to radiation and ignorant that radiation injury to the arteries is delayed as long as 10 years.

Radiation has its only role at the end game. It can provide brilliant palliation for distressing local symptoms such as bleeding in the bladder. Twenty-six of 29 patients irradiated for late stage symptoms about the bladder neck unresponsive to hormone deprivation were symptom free at three years. Only 10-20% of patients near to death from prostate cancer experience debilitating symptoms from the primary site of the cancer. This late use of radiation for palliation represents a small market and so is not advertised in the *Sunday Times Magazine*. The profit margin due to volume in the worried well is far greater and so the worried well are pursued.

Radium-223 is an alpha particle emitter. The alpha particle has a very short trajectory and so does not fry the rest of the bone marrow. It is approved for payment in the United States under Medicare because it has lengthened cancer-specific life significantly. This therapy should be used in the case of a bone marrow aspirate positive for prostate cancer cells, whose bone scan is nonetheless negative for cancer deposits big enough to be read as a positive bone scan. That would be truly early systemic therapy.

CHAPTER 10

The systemic nature of prostate cancer: the detection of cancer cells in circulating blood, bone marrow, and lymph nodes by molecular means.

"That tumor growth and progression is limited before vascularization of the neoplastic mass is generally accepted. Vascularization is achieved via neoangiogenesis, co-option of existing blood vessels, vasculogenic mimcry (in which poorly differentiated, highly malignant tumor cells can form a primitive vascular system), or a combination of these processes."[322] "Disseminated tumor cells were detected (in bone marrow) in 74% (395/537) of patients prior to radical prostatectomy."[1a]

"This article by Mejean and Associates emphasizes the value of RT-PCR for PSA in predicting treatment outcome in patients for localized disease." Carl Olson, M.D. Professor and Chairman, Dept. of Urology, College of Physicians and Surgeons of Columbia University, New York, New York.[323]

In the late 1930s, A.R. Rich, a pathologist, told U.S. urologists that the smallest, occult cancers found incidentally at autopsy had metastasized to the lymphatics channels adjacent to the nerves in the prostate 30% of the time with one slice through the prostate. This work was repeated in 2004 and identical metastases were found to be present in 79% of radical prostatectomy specimens using a quotidian staining technique.[324] I believe that special monoclonal antibody staining would change that to 100%. Moreover, lymphatics around nerve sheaths are not where prostate cancer cells thrive. Since the nineteenth century, prostate cancer has been known to thrive selectively in bone marrow.[325,326] Data on doubling times to be presented in a later chapter show that androgen deprivation has half the effect on the cancer in the bone marrow that it has on cancer in lymph nodes. This is why patients die of rampant prostate cancer growth in their marrow while the cancer in the nodes adds up to less damage. Second year medical students learn about prostate cancer's predeliction for marrow during their course in pathology.

Philosophers of science tell us that the burden of proof falls on the person who claims something exists. In this case, how do we know that metastases exist in the bone marrow prior to radical surgery, radiotherapy, freezing or any other focal modality that pretends to "get it all"? During my 1969-1973 urology residency at Columbia Presbyterian Medical Center in N.Y.C., we routinely drew bone marrow specimens from the superior iliac spine of patients with prostate cancer to be tested for prostatic acid phosphatase, an early marker for prostate cancer. If the marrow level was higher than the peripheral blood, radical surgery was canceled. By the mid-1970s, reports about a biochemical check for metastases in the bone marrow in candidates for focal therapy to the primary site disappeared from our journals.

It was not until 1986, just after the development of prostate specific antigen (PSA), that publications about bone marrow aspirations reappeared. Patients with nuclear bone scans negative for metastases were once **again** shown to have metastases by aspiration of the marrow itself and then by treatment of the aspirate with sensitive, PSA staining.[327] Two years later, in 1988, just as the epidemic of radical surgery was beginning to heat up, supersensitive, highly specific stains again showed metastases to be commonly present in the bone marrow of persons with no sign of metastases in the marrow by nuclear scan.[328] That is over twenty years before this book!

Five years later, in 1993, a year after the peak of the epidemic of surgery in the elderly, approximately one third of patients who would otherwise qualify for surgery for putative cure were shown to have cancer cells in their marrow by a technique of staining with monoclonal antibodies.[329] This technique was far simpler than the older technique reported above. The older technique using messenger RNA amplification was so tricky that its use by the prosecution resulted in O.J. Simpson's exoneration. The monoclonal antibody data was quickly confirmed in August of 1994 by a group from Memorial-Sloan Kettering Hospital in N.Y.C. In their study, two out of nine patients with a negative conventional pre-radical prostatectomy workup for metastases showed prostate cancer cells in their marrow.[330] Again in 1994, in a much larger series of bone marrow aspirates from eighty-nine patients, 33% stained positive for cytokeratin-18, a chemical group characteristic of cells derived from glands of which prostate is an example.[331] Cytokeratin-18 has no proper business in bone marrow. A third of those positive for cytokeratin-18 also stained for prostate specific antigen (PSA). Control patients, those without known cancer, were negative. Thus, by 1994 in my opinion, it was impossible to say that prostate cancer nodules in excess of two millimeters in diameter had not metastasized. After 1994, metastases to the marrow should have been a mandatory inference by a prudent man. Every time a more sensitive test for cancer in the marrow was devised, more citizens turned out to have metastatic disease at an earlier stage. By 1994 it was clear to serious students of the disease that all persons with clinically significant cancer in the prostate had metastases far from the original site and that extended resection of uninvolved tissues in the primary site would not prolong life as it had not in the case of breast cancer.

Like all medical tests, these tests of the bone marrow aspirate are neither perfectly sensitive nor perfectly specific. For example, we were cautioned in 1994 that a negative test for cytokeratin-18 in the marrow does not mean that there are no metastases. In science we say the "absence of evidence is not evidence of absence." All cancer cells tend to make more and more errors in the DNA as time passes. In so doing, they lose, as we saw in the case of infant neuroblastoma, the characteristic chemicals on their surface that say they are from, in the case of neuroblastoma, nerve cell progenitors. In the case of cytokeratin-18, such a loss occurs in 50% of a wide range of cancers, including prostate, metastatic to marrow.[332] A bone marrow aspiration which does not stain for cytokeratin-18 or PSA does not mean you are out of the woods. It may even mean you are deeper into the woods because the cancer has become too primitive to express this molecule on its surface.

But the data keeps getting stronger for the intrinsically metastatic nature of prostate cancer, if that were needed after the observations of the 1930s. By 2000, 85% of **pre**-radical prostatectomy patients had been reported to be positive for disseminated prostate cancer cells in the marrow when the monoclonal antibodies were tagged with iron and concentrated with a magnet.[333] When a second bone marrow was aspirated **after** radical prostatectomy because of a rising prostate specific antigen, 83% were still positive! In a study from the same group with the same concentrating technique three years later, we find that 90% of their patients before radical prostatectomy show epithelial cells in their marrow.[334] A 2004 report from the same group says that PSA positivity in the bone marrow by enriched immunohistochemistry correlated strongly with early recurrence.[335] As we might expect from the 1994 warning about the loss of specific surface chemicals as cancer cells become more and more primitive, only 60% of these cells expressed the prostate specific antigen (PSA). Only one of 20 control patients showed epithelial cells in the marrow. The one was a man over 50 and he could have had an occult adenocarcinoma somewhere, even prostate cancer. This same test, with its clever concentration of cells by magnetic forces on iron particles, should eventually be commercially available from Immunicon of Huntington Valley, P.A.[336] It should be payable by Medicare for prostate cancer because it correlates with clinical outcome and would cancel thousands of radical surgeries and radiation attempts.[337] A similar system using the CellSearch system and an EpCAM antibody for cells in the peripheral blood has been approved for predicting progression free and overall survival in prostate cancer.[338]

It is important to note that the authors of University of Washington studies did not conclude that a proposed radical prostatectomy should be scrubbed when prostate cancer cells have been identified in the marrow. They argued, instead, that because none of the patients had died of prostate cancer five years after surgery, their findings should not be used in the argument against radical surgery. But my published figure for the **mean** time to death is 17.5 years for these early, non-palpable cancers; the University of Washington figure of five years of follow up is less than one quarter of the way to the **median** time to death at 22 years. The authors say that "these cells are present in men who will not develop clinical evidence of disease for many years…" That is true but it is also true that these men are not cured, in the plain meaning of that word, by resection of the primary site. If they had known that pre-operatively, they might not have consented to radical surgery which implies cure.

Another claim by those who would continue radiation and radical surgery as usual is that all these cells in the marrow die. Undoubtedly, many do. It has been known since the 1970s via cell kinetic studies that as many as 90% of the cells of a cancer, even at its primary site, may die. The laboratories at Columbia's P&S were very important in the discovery of apoptosis, cell suicide in cancer. Without question, metastases have an even harder time getting a foothold. An expert on metastases has estimated that only ".1% of cells reaching the target organ parenchyma go on to form metastases."[339] But .1% of millions of cells over fourteen years means hundreds of metastatic sites all growing exponentially.

Minute numbers of specific cells can be identified by looking for the messenger RNA responsible for the manufacture of the cell's known products, in this case PSA. This was the technique used in the attempted conviction of O.J. Simpson. It is fussy and prone to error. That is the reason the jury did not convict. The first report of metastatic prostate cancer cells identified by the O.J. technique in the blood of those undergoing radical prostatectomy came from my alma mater, Columbia's College of Physicians and Surgeons in New York, again in the critical year, 1994.[340] It was shown to be true even after biopsy.[341] The apologists for extensive local therapy dismiss this data on the grounds that it has not been correlated with clinical deterioration. But it has. In fact, the presence of circulating prostate cancer cells was correlated with clinical deterioration in the following year, 1995,[342] and confirmed in 1996[343] and 2001.[344] The most recent Columbia report, supported by grants from the New York Academy of Medicine, the Koch Foundation, the T.J. Martell Foundation and the National Cancer Institute, correlated outcome with the presence of circulating prostate cancers after radiotherapy as well.[345] They found circulating cells to be a sign of poor prognosis. Their findings after radiotherapy were confirmed most recently in 2003 by a group at the United States Armed Forces Medical School who concentrated the cancer cells circulating in the blood with a magnet, the Immunicon technique. They found 83% of their prostate cancer patients have such cells.[346]

The Columbia University group, the first to announce the detection of circulating prostate cancer cells via the messenger RNA amplification technique, said they were going to develop a reference lab. That has not happened. Stephen Kaplan, M.D., of the Department of Urology at Columbia told me that the technique proved too fussy to transfer to a commercial reference lab[347] and so it is not payable by Medicare. That is a business of medicine issue, not a scientific one.

There is no monetary reinforcement for a test that proves the systemic nature of prostate cancer in the United States. It is not an accident that recent research on the MGA-E gene regarding the correlation of positive findings in the marrow with clinic deterioration comes from the socialized medicine of Germany on a grant from the Cancer Research Institute of New York. But the practical effect is that the many publications cited above have not yet affected practice, even of the university departments of urology responsible. Maybe this book will change that.

Instead of aspirating the bone marrow, where prostate cancer thrives but nobody gets paid, the specialties of urology and radiology have spent the last twenty years chasing lymph nodes, where prostate cancer does not dwell readily, but where each specialty is well paid for imaging techniques or biopsies. Representative of current research is an elegant recent demonstration that prostate cancer metastases to lymph nodes can be identified by scanning the patient with magnetic resonance imaging (MRI) after intravenous injection of lymphotropic superparamagnetic nanoparticles.[348] A report about this test caused a serious spike in the relevant stock. Like other tests, this one is useful when its sensitivity threshold is exceeded but tells us nothing when it is not. Moreover, as above, lymph nodes are not the favored residence of prostate cancer cells. The marrow is. Nobody cares. You can make money chasing lymph nodes because they are often negative in this disease. There is no money in aspirating marrow, only money to be lost by positively proving metastatic disease. The loss is caused by the cancellation of radical surgery or focal radiation for alleged cure.

CHAPTER 11

Medical castration prolongs life.

In 1962, the Department of Physiology at Columbia's College of Physicians and Surgeons (known as P&S) in the city of New York required each second year medical student to write a review of a physiologic topic. I submitted a review of the releasing factors at the base of the brain which travel one centimeter down to the pituitary via specialized vessels and cause it to release its hormones. I chose this topic because my grandfather, John Rogers, P&S 1892, had been one of New York's first surgical endocrinologists. My mother described him as taking tadpoles in a bucket to their weekend house in Towners, N.Y., to feed them thyroid extract. When I was about nine, she gave me a book of human anatomy for my birthday (part of her plot to make me want to be an M.D.) which showed the pituitary as a command center in royal purple. I decided at that time to be an endocrinologist.

In the summer of 1962, after my first year of medical school, I asked A.V. Schally, Ph.D., and R. Guillemin, M.D., Ph.D. at Baylor University's new facility in the Texas Medical Center in Houston for a summer job in their lab. The lab was concerned with the structure of corticotrophin releasing factor (CRF). CRF traveled from the hypothalamus of the brain to the pituitary via the venous system and caused it to release adrenocortiocotrophin hormone (ACTH). My grandfather, clinical professor of surgery at N.Y. Cornell, knew nothing of these releasing factors.[349] This, in turn, caused the release of one of the stress response hormones from the adrenal glands. It seemed to me that the structure of CRF was the important question because once you were able to synthesize the peptide, there would be plenty of material and, therefore, time to do physiologic experiments. A scientist in England, G.W. Harris, had been frittering away the minute amounts of CRF he could obtain naturally on physiologic experiments. That seemed to me a poor idea.

A.V. Schally accepted my presence in the lab after reading my review for the physiology department at P&S. I drove to Houston in June when some of my classmates were becoming lifeguards. My assignment was to learn how the talented laboratory technician, Surlina Robinson, did the bioassays designed by Dr. Guillemin for CRF activity of the extracts of brain delivered from Schally's lab. I was to do the bioassays when she went on vacation. This was blue collar work. I was in no sense a scientist but I did become facile in the lab which was my goal. Surlina and I would go down in the basement to block the release of corticotrophin-releasing hormone from the base of the brains of rats (the hypothalamus) with a combination of morphine and phenobarbital. We created two peacefully dozing white rows of rodents under the influence of ether. Sometimes I became drowsy too because of the ether. After a half hour, we would then inject them with one of Dr. Guillemin's biologicals, at that time, mostly posterior pituitary extract, wait a while, then sacrifice them and draw blood for cortisol, one of the stress response hormones from the adrenal. We were getting very little cortisol release from the posterior pituitary extract biological.

Dr. Guillemin was to leave for France, where he had a second laboratory, in early July, 1962. Just before he left, he called me into his office to become better acquainted with me. He said that he had read a paper the previous night by S. M. McCann of the University of Pennsylvania on luteinizing hormone releasing factor (LHRF). He said that McCann had "scooped" him. He repeated the word "scooped" twice and appeared proud of his American vernacular. The Schally-Guillemin use of McCann's report was the origin of vast pharmaceutical fortunes which cost Medicare as much money as all urological operations combined in 2003. The combined average profit from injecting the resultant medicine, Lupron or Zoladex (LHRF agonists-antagonists), for a year in a typical urology practice could be as much as $94, 847,[350] a figure now, as I write, under vigorous downward revision by the Medicare administration. Japanese urologists in private practice made similar profits on the administration of this class of drugs until recently.[351]

In August, when it seemed as though Houston would spontaneously combust moments before it drowned in the afternoon thunderstorms, Dr. Schally went on a holiday to Florida, Surlina went to her home in Tyler, Texas, and I went down to the Houston packing plant in one hundred degree heat. I stood beside a Mexican worker devoid of English who was harvesting pituitaries from hog skulls. I would cut out the hypothalamus, a square area at the base of the brain. This went on for two weeks. When Dr. Schally returned, he was thrilled to see vat after vat of hypothalami in his freezers. To me the two weeks with the hogs were a small price to pay to become facile in the lab.

Thus, the topic of interruption of the brain pituitary axis is not something I read in a book, but something I have lived. I have held the hypothalamus, the source of luteinizing hormone releasing factor (LHRF), in my hand hundreds of times. I saw the chemical columns used to isolate it that had just been imported from Sweden by Dr. Guillemin. Prof. Schally and Dr. Guillemin were given the Nobel Prize in 1977 for the structure of LHRF. They had moved to separate labs and engaged in a fifteen year competition for the structure as described in Nicholas Wade's book, *The Nobel Duel.*[352, 353] The science of hypothalamic releasing factors has expanded prodigiously since then. It turns out that these factors and their receptors are located all over and do a lot besides releasing pituitary hormones as described in a review provided to me recently by Dr. Guillemin.[354]

About 1932, before superagonists based on the structure of LHRF were used in the 1990s to lower male hormone in prostate cancer, castration for prostate cancer started.[355] An isolated case of improvement was published by the Mayo Clinic in 1936.[356] Hugh Young, the originator of the radical procedure for prostate cancer as described earlier, made a visit to the clinic in this period in an attempt to sell his radical prostatectomy. Young made no sale to Mayo. I surmise that some early success of castration for cancer, which had been done since the mid-nineteenth century for BPH, gave the clinic a medical alternative.

These early anecdotal reports about the relief afforded by lowering the male hormone were more firmly grounded in science[357] by Huggins of the University of Chicago in 1941. He showed that acid phosphatase, an enzyme made by prostate cancer cells, declined when the male hormone level was lowered via the negative feed back of estrogen administration or castration. *Per contra*, the serum acid phosphatase level increased with the administration of male hormone.[358] Castration and/or the administration of female hormone produced, after 1941, an immediate life extension of about three years as seen in the survival curves I have abstracted from the Ann Arbor, Michigan, urology clinic pre- and post World War II. See Figure 1.

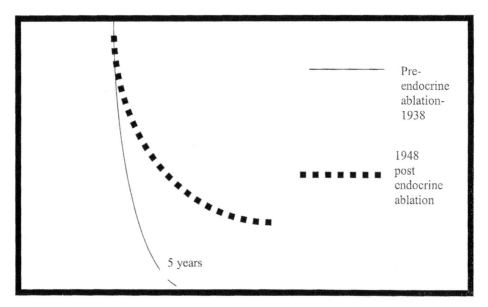

FIGURE 1

Percent survival after first presentation to the urology clinic at the University of Michigan before and after the discovery of the efficacy of androgen ablation.

After Huggins' work had publicity, 5 year survival increased about 30%. There were rare long term cures in which it appeared that every cancer cell required testosterone to live and, conversely, that every cancer cell died when deprived of it.

The next critical event in the story of androgen deprivation was the 1973 report by the Veterans Administration that the estrogens at the customary 3 mg/ day dose given to lower the levels of male hormones, measurably increased deaths due to heart attack and strokes.[359] I believed it. In the late 1970s, during my private practice days in Manhattan, one of my patients was admitted to the hospital with pressing substernal chest pain one day after I had started him on estrogen. A second patient was admitted with a thrombosis of his leg a few days after I started estrogen. An extensive literature developed which showed that certain proteins that promote clotting increase with this 3 mg. dose of estrogen. I have only given it when the patient could afford nothing else since then.

During the period after estrogen's harmful effect at three milligrams was revealed, but before Lupron (an LHRF agonist/antagonist) was approved, it was the urologist's unpleasant job to ask for the patient's testicles instead. One of the residents in my residency program in a city hospital in New York was told on the telephone by a patient's son that, if he "took off my daddy's testicles," that the son would come and kill the doctor. During my time at the Veterans Administration in Walla Walla, Washington, a patient came in with terrible bone pain from cancer of the prostate. The private sector had stripped him of his money in false attempts to "get it all." I did a castration because the chief of staff had taken Lupron off the pharmacy list to save money (even though the pharmacy was within its budget). The morning after I did his surgical castration the patient did not feel relief of his bone pain. Disappointed, he took decisive action in the way of the United States far west. He took a gun out of his luggage and shot himself in the head as he lay in the hospital bed moments before I arrived for morning rounds. V.A. regulations require that all luggage be searched for guns but such a search was not performed in this case. There was blood everywhere. He could have shot me or one of the nurses.

Tempers run high about castration. Exactly how androgen is to be lowered in this disease is, therefore, not academic onanism. In this instance, we literally hear the "sound of the guns" that military boards require for promotion and I claim as part of the platform for this book.

Patient mishaps like that above caused the specialty of urology to greet with joyous huzzas FDA approval in 1994 of Lupron, an analogue agonist/antagonist of Schally and Guillimen's releasing hormone. It meant we did not have to surgically castrate anybody anymore. Nor did we run the risk of being shot or of causing heart attacks and strokes with oral estrogen. Lupron took the testosterone to zero in a month by occupying binding sites in the pituitary. It used to cost about $2,000 for a shot that lasted three months currently. There is no way to justify that cost as compared to the cost of surgical orchiectomy except on psychological grounds.

But cost was no problem to the Medicare administration in the early days. The legislation, as passed in 1966, created a tragedy of the commons wherein nobody cared about cost particularly when the word cancer was involved. The males of the United States, including Prof. Max Lerner during its pre-FDA approval stage, as described in the chapter on the humanist response, chose a reversible medical castration over an irreversible surgical castration every time. Sales at TAP Pharmaceuticals of Lupron rose from 550 million in 1995 to 4000 million in 2000.[360] The latter figure was a far greater cost than all the urological procedures combined under Medicare. This enthusiasm among urologists occurred, not only because of the persistent drum beat of evidence that androgen deprivation lengthens life when given early, but also because the Medicare administration reimbursed urologists hundreds of dollars more than the cost of acquisition.

A second reason to avoid surgical castration emerged in the late 1990s, from the urology department at the University of B.C., Vancouver. They showed that intermittent androgen deprivation was just as good as continuous deprivation. This was a discovery that could have been made at any time since 1941 but just was not investigated. The discovery of the doubling time of prostate cancer to be 475 days in 1995 tells us that a year and a half of deprivation is enough. At that point, presumably all the cells that need testosterone to avoid programmed cell death, apoptosis, should be dead. In addition to that rationale, there is reason to believe that neighboring, dedicated fibroblasts in the prostate, when re-exposed to testosterone, exert a disciplinary action on the cancer cells and cause some of them to be less invasive. If the testicles remain, they may return male hormones to the patient later without the expensive intramuscular injections of male hormones every other week. The inexpensive oral preparation sometimes poisons the liver. Men have more initiative when their male hormones are at normal levels. That is more important with the self employed.

Most recently, a pill, not an injection, called Casodex that blocks the action of male hormones out at the tissue receptor level has been shown to prolong evidence of recurrence when given early. In other words, the postman brings the mail but cannot put it in the mailbox because it is stuffed full of earlier, spurious deliveries. Casodex costs $350.00 for one month, too much for my patients. Businessmen call this opportunity pricing.

Two issues remain hot, as I write, in regard to lowering the male hormone for cancer control. The first issue is whether early androgen deprivation actually lengthens life. If prostate cancer is considered to be an exponential function like the compound interest of your savings account, you get three years of extra life after the standard 80% kill of cancer cells caused by androgen deprivation. Mathematically, it does not matter whether you do it early or late because it is a distributive function. But here the mathematics conflict with the data in the Dunning R 3327 model. There, the earlier castration is performed, the longer the rat lives, e.g. his life is extended from 350 days to 475 days or 42% if the castration is done the day of tumor implantation.[361] For every 50 days delay in castration, the rat loses approximately 50 days of life. Applied to man, i.e.

42% of the 17.5 years mean time to death from the sort of cancer discovered by PSA, this means androgen ablation at the time of discovery should add about 7.3 years of life.[362] Three studies in man have supported that supposition.[363,364,365] A man was reported to have responded for 27 years to androgen ablation therapy after presenting with multiple metastatic spots on his nuclear bone scan.[366] When he finally showed metastases on his bone scan again, he responded to a chemotherapeutic poison plus a modern LHRF agonist-antagonist.

Data from Japan supports the mathematical prediction and the anecdote above. Of 176 patients with radical prostatectomy plus androgen deprivation, 11% died of prostate cancer within 10 years while 11.2% of 151 patients with androgen ablation **alone** died of prostate cancer within 10 years.[367] This was not a statistically significant difference. **Radical prostatectomy contributed nothing that was not gained by androgen deprivation alone**. But there is something even more interesting about this series. The series was prospective but not randomized. The androgen deprivation series without radical prostatectomy was, on average, 8.5 years older and therefore 8.5 years **deeper into the natural history of the disease**. Because of this there should have been 11.5 extra deaths in the series of androgen alone or, alternatively, there should have been 11.5 fewer deaths in the surgical wing. In this series, **radical surgery for prostate cancer appears to have hastened the time to death**. One of the chief investigators of the Japanese study agreed with this interpretation via email.[368] Acceleration of cancer specific death by radical surgery is not surprising to me. I have reported the acceleration of cancer death by radical surgery for muscle invasive bladder cancer at the V.A. in Fresno, CA, in a peer reviewed venue. Modern cancer cell biology predicts it through diminution of cell suicide.

The Japanese series was accepted as a discussed poster at the American Urological Association (A.U.A.) meeting in Atlanta, Georgia, 2006. Its acceptance for discussion signals that one A.U.A. committee member was not content with the chop and/or burn approach to primary site of prostate cancer care. A poster acceptance is the camel's nose under the medical/political tent.

But you get nothing for free in the cancer business. A low testosterone, hypogonadism, is a disease. My grandfather, Columbia P&S 1892, lived long enough to see supplementary testosterone and knew its value. The epidemic of prostate cancer diagnosis and care created a vast, unprecedented, and for a long time unrecorded, population of hypogonadal males for two reasons: (1) 30-60% of the radical prostatectomy specimens show cancer at the margins. In essence, the radical prostatectomy sold as curative, is really a lumpectomy similar to that now done for breast cancer to determine the severity of disease but not to cure it. The "I think I got it all" ploy is immediately exposed as fraudulent by margin positivity. The cancer is then reclassified as systemic, a reason to cause hypogonadism with intensely profitable Lupron shots given in the office. (2) As recorded by Max Lerner, the cultural critic, and George Sheehan, the M.D. runner, in their books about their prostate cancers in the next chapter, LHRF agonists-antagonists created an alternative to surgical castration, a tough psychological wound. Lupron and Zoladex became billion dollar businesses.

In the resulting swirl of commerce, Lupron caused a number of urologists to come to legal and regulatory grief when they sold pricey vials to patients and ultimately to Medicare which they had obtained for free as samples. TAP pharmaceuticals gave them the free samples as part of an intense competition with AstraZeneca's agonist-antagonist called Zoladex, a slightly different pharmacologic formulation of the agonist-antagonist Lupron concept. AstraZeneca's sales of Zoladex increased 16% for the nine months of 2002 from $519 million to $595 million. The latter figure is small beer in the report of this vast corporation whose real money comes from Prilosec at sales of 3.6 billion dollars for the nine months of 2002.[369] The stock, if purchased in 1998, would have doubled your money by 2003, if you take note of the split in mid-1998. This would have been good work in the dot com stock market bust. TAP Pharmaceuticals has been accused of manipulating its wholesale price for Lupron knowing that Medicare bases its reimbursement rates on that price.

Because early androgen deprivation was both profitable and biologically wise, the epidemic of radical surgery has mutated into an epidemic of osteoporosis. I showed a poster on this topic to the annual meeting of the Western Section of the American Urological Association in 1994.[370] The chairman and professor of Urology at the University of British Columbia, Lorne D. Sullivan, M.D., who mediated the poster session, thanked me during a social event later for bringing up osteoporosis as a complication and Didronel and diphosphonate as the solution. This is how scientific medicine proceeds, by posters attended by a person, by a podium presentation, a word here, a word there, and personal contact at a meeting. It does not proceed via journal articles.

Fortunately, the osteoporosis of hypogonadism can be prevented by diphosphonates, another costly/profitable group of drugs depending on who is paying, which may even have direct anti-prostate cancer activity in the bone marrow. Less well documented but as important are the changes in cognitive function that follow hypogonadism. Recall for words is cut in half while executive ability is improved. President Clinton, if given one of the anti-androgren drugs well before his inauguration, would have made shorter speeches and thought more about his future. Despite these drawbacks, the serious life extension described above, plus the serious profits possible via office injection have combined to create a vast androgen ablation market.

Yet another effect of the castrate state is prolongation of the repolarization of the heart after the normal wave of conduction passes through. This effect is not as great if a pure antagonist such as Degarelix Acetate (generic) or Firmagon (commercial) is used than if the older generation of agonist-antagonists is used with a peripheral androgen blocker. The effect was a small but significant increase of 13 to 18 milleseconds in a total of 402 milleseconds, something for those with heart disease to think about.[371]

Many of these complications may be avoidable with a shorter course. Even a 6 month induction of androgen suppression may extend life as much as the 2 to 3 years of continuous suppression can.[372] Nothing is written in stone about this 65-year-old topic. It is hot.

CHAPTER 12

The growth of prostate cancer as an exponential function: why it is often so slow.

"Calculus differs from these subjects (elementary algebra) in that it stresses another operation, that of taking a limit."[373]

While English is fair at conveying truth, mathematics is better. The reader must take himself/herself back to high school and contemplate once again the miracle of compound interest working on his savings account or, in the case before us, cancer of the prostate. Coffey and Isaacs of Johns Hopkins first published these calculations in 1979.[374] At that time, the doubling time for other common killer cancers had been established to be about 58 days.[375] Using the formula for compound interest, Coffey and Isaacs calculated that at such a growth rate "it would take four years for one cell to grow to the size of a match head" and an additional 2.5 years to grow to 2 pounds, or one liter, stipulated by oncologists to be a fatal burden. These are the times we see for the common killers, breast and lung. Pancreas is quicker at three to five months.

Coffey and Isaacs were employed by the Department of Urology at Johns Hopkins and so suspected that the doubling time for prostate cancer was longer than 58 days. But the longest doubling time they explored in their calculations was 365 days. At that rate, it would be 25 years from the critical DNA error to .03 cubic centimeters that would allow identification as cancer with a microscope. A 365 day doubling time also implies 15 years from the first true positive identification with a microscope to death, and a 40 year total time from incipience to death at one thousand cubic centimeters of cancer.

Coffey and Isaacs, in 1979, underestimated the sluggishness of prostate cancer. Sixteen years later, in 1995, this same Johns Hopkins group measured the actual doubling time using immunocytochemistry on human cancers. It turned out, at 475 days plus or ± 56 days, to be 25% longer than they had envisioned years earlier. It is that slow because this cancer has a proclivity toward cell suicide that almost equals, at certain sites, its mitotic rate. This longer doubling time implied a fifty-two year natural history from the first fully cancerous cell to death, and thirty-nine and a half years to achieve a tumor diameter of one centimeter, big enough to feel with a digital rectal examination. When thirty-nine years is subtracted from the mean age of diagnosis, seventy-two years, we learn that most prostate cancers, to be fatal, must start early in the third decade of life, way before current screening programs begin.

Note well that the Hopkins group found quicker growth rates in the metastatic sites. The doubling time in lymph nodes was thirty-three days, about twice as fast as in bone marrow and fourteen times as fast as in the primary site. The absence of male hormone also made a big difference. It slowed the growth in lymph nodes by a factor of four and in marrow only by a factor of two. That is why metastases in the bone marrow dominate the last days in this disease and not lymph node disease. They all have been deprived of testosterone when the metastases could be seen on a nuclear bone scan.

The implications of the Coffey and Isaacs approach to prostate cancer as an exponential function are not obvious until two more dates in the progress of the cancer are placed on the graph.[376] They are: (1) the mean time to death for incidental, occult prostate cancer at 17.5 ± 1.8 years, my data published in the British Journal of Urology in 2000[377]; (2) the time at which a developing sphere of cells begins to metastasize, 1-2 millimeters.[378] It may be half that.

To facilitate your grasp of a four hundred and seventy five day doubling time, let us interpret the first prostate cancer cell as a deposit to a savings account subject to compound interest. (1) The "principle" has a "value" of .000000001 cubic centimeters, the volume of a single cell; (2) The doubling time of four hundred and seventy-five days translates into an annual interest rate of 76%; (3) Death occurs when the account reaches a volume of 1000 cubic centimeters; (4) Metastases occur at 2 millimeters or .00314cc's, maybe much less and much earlier; (5) The average volume of cancer in radical prostatectomy specimens taken from a man with a PSA less than 4.0 ug/dl is 2.5 centimeters;[379] (6) The mean time to death from incidental occult cancer is 17.5 years as above; (7) Androgen ablation kills 80% of the cells.

The Visa card compound interest rate calculator on the internet[380] yields the following results with regard to time given the six assumptions above. The volume of the primary cancer becomes the hands on a biological clock so that we can read the time. The cancer that can kill you starts at age 30-40. Metastases begin 28.5 years into the natural history when a volume of .004 cc's is reached, a diameter of 2 millimeters, about age 58-68. See Figure 1.

Incidental, occult carcinomas are discovered at transurethral resection of BPH or by PSA directed biopsy at a volume of .116 ccs after 6.5 years of metastatic showers in the blood stream and lymphatics. Radical prostatectomy commonly occurs at 2.5 centimeters (from the graph) forty years into the natural history and (from the graph) after **twelve years of metastatic showers**. Death occurs, without androgen ablation, in the fifty-second year after the formation of the first true cancer cell. Androgen ablation, by

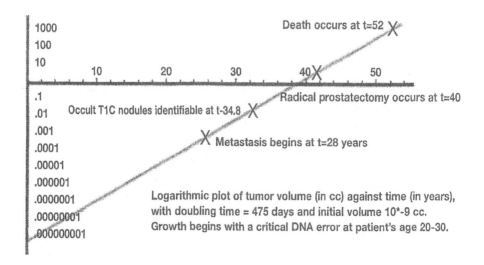

FIGURE 1

Prostate cancer depicted as an exponential function on semilog paper with an annual interest rate of 76%. Radical prostatectomy typically occurs after 12 years of metastases. This operation does not 'cure.' Both the Swedish and V.A. series show no difference between surgery and observation at 15 and 10 years. This appeared as a poster at the annual meeting of the Western Section of the A.U.A., Nov. 1st, 2003, at Las Vegas, NV.

depriving 80% of the cells of immortality resets the clock back three years. It adds three years of life. Mathematically you get the three years whether androgen ablation is done early or late because it is a distributive function according to this paradigm. This mathematical result conflicts with the biological evidence in animals and man that early androgen deprivation extends life more than late. The median time to death after radical prostatectomy plus androgen ablation in node positive patients is more than 15 years after the operation,[381] the time predicted in 1979 by Coffey and Isaacs for their maximal, theoretical, three hundred and sixty five day, doubling time.

What would be the effect of removing the 2.5 cc's of cancer in the prostate, the average volume according to the Stanford group, according to the mathematics? In the forty-second year of life of the cancer, one can read off the graph a gain of 1.5 years via radical prostatectomy.

This result is gratifyingly close to the 9-20 months of life gained through radical prostatectomy according to computer modeling of screening detected populations aged 65 years[382] and better than the one month predicted in the study of Proscar as a preventive measure. Thus, radical prostatectomy probably does yield a little extra time on this earth but it is less than 1.8 years, one standard deviation of the mean time to death from an incidental cancer. Thus, if the patient did live an extra year and a half, he would never know whether it was the operation or a roll of the dice that was responsible. Thus, neither radical surgery nor nerve sparing cryosurgery, which I championed as an alternative, can be proven to lengthen life in the sense of the enlightenment.

The objection is often made that probabilities are not useful in the individual clinical case. Such was the response of John Isaacs, Ph.D. to an editorial I published July of 2000 in the American Urological Association News urging my specialty to tell their patients the age of their prostate cancers at discovery.[383] Instead, Prof. Isaacs proposed a not yet commercially available assay of each individual cancer's doubling time in a dish. My reply to his proposal is that we M.D.s use aggregate probabilities in our most quotidian decisions. Here, what he considers best would be a serious enemy of the good because in essence it is a plea for the status quo. Individual assays are not available. That gives us license to continue to ignore what we do know. Also, an individual assay might be seriously misleading because doubling times in a dish are very different from those at various locations in the body where the cancer cells are subject to the discipline of neighboring fibroblasts. Fibroblasts are the skeleton of the soft tissues and have the job of regulating the growth of their more specialized neighbors via messenger molecules called cytokines.

It is incorrect for the public to assume that medical care decisions are made with perfect information. This is not possible in the stock market nor in my business. Both sectors stumble into the future through a fog of probabilities. Andy Grove in his article in Fortune magazine about his choice of radioactive seeds was very keen on the enumeration of his probabilities. By now, most of the new investors drawn into the stock market in the last decade have learned that certainties do not exist in that arena. With that hard lesson, they should have little difficulty with the metaphor of the original prostate cancer cell as a deposit earning compound interest of about 76% per year.

A weakness of the model is the fact that the mean time to death should be less than seventeen years because of the faster (150 days) doubling times of metastases than at the primary site. My explanation for the delay is that many of the cells must commit suicide when they leave the dedicated fibroblasts at the primary site. Under normal circumstances at their home base, fibroblasts dedicated to the prosperity of the prostate, like a friendly policeman talking to a potential suicide on a bridge, encourage the cancer cells not to do it. When the cancer cells leave home base, the policemen are not so friendly; the cancer cells do commit suicide in large numbers, and the growth of the tumor nodule slows.

To some this model is too intellectual but I ask, "What is the alternative? Throw up your hands and make no statement about what the future holds at all?" This has, in fact, been the practice in my specialty. In fact a letter in response to my article in the British Journal of Urology about the mean time to death from incidentally discovered prostate cancer urged just that. Two British doctors said it was better to do no calculations at all and continue to gull the public. The public does like the concealment of what we do know. They are used to a time line in the strategic planning of their businesses and they want one for their life span under various treatment scenarios.

CHAPTER 13

Humanists report on their experience with prostate cancer.

U rology and radiation oncology, in my opinion, need an audit committee made up of outside directors in the matter of prostate cancer discovery and treatment. Kurt Goedel proved in the 1930s that formal systems cannot audit themselves insofar as they are formal. This paradox was known to the ancient Greeks as the problem of the meaning of "All Cretans are Liars," when spoken by a man from Crete. Goedel proved that the sentence was content-free even though it looks like language. This is why we have outside directors for major corporations who will speak up loudly. For lack of dissenting voice, General Motors failed to reform itself, as Toyota did, in anticipation of a leap in the price of oil. I nominate in this chapter for outside directors in the proposed audit committee, humanists who have experienced prostate cancer and bothered to write a book about it. In my view, an author looks at his subject with the same prolonged intensity as the scientist but uses less mathematics to represent his perceptions.

There are six worthy accounts by professional writers of their experience with prostate cancer. A common thread is their attitude towards time. How much time do they imagine inhabiting the earth without prostate cancer and how much with it? Some time issues are tabulated below in Table 1.

Oliver Sacks, in his foreword to Broyard's book quoted him as saying, "the threat of dying ought to make people witty." This is the opposite of a call for a stop watch, measuring tape, scales, and the latest PSA value. Science is not typically thought of as a witty enterprise but it can be. Flashes of insight can bind disparate observations together, much like a good joke. Dr. Sacks saw the natural outcome of Broyard's witty death as a wish for a physician "...who is not only a talented physician, but a bit of a metaphysician too...."[384] He asks for more than my specialty can typically give routinely.[385]

Broyard's wife, in her foreword, points out the magical thinking involved. He believed, she wrote, "...that he could outwit his cancer by constructing an alternative

Author	Intrinsic Metastatic Nature Mentioned by Consultants	Ca stage	Treatment	Comments	Age	Meta Comment	Presented As	Lived After Diagnosis
Broyard, Intoxicated by My Illness	N.A.	8/89, Given 6 to 18 months.	Estrogen; Search for immortality through personal style.	Wanted a humanist urologist; appreciated his mortality for the first time.	69	No grade but it must have been a Gleason 8 or above.	Retention	1.16 years
Cornelius Ryan Professional Writer	No	D1, pos. Lympnan-giogram 1970	Iodine seeds, writing a book endocrine, chemo' late	Unrealistic about speed of disease	50	Grade not given. Musc.	Prostatitis with retention.	4.5 years
M. Korda, Book editor. Man to Man	No	T2-T3, 9/94	Rad. surg.	Morbidity Cognitive	60	6	PSA 25 BPH	>10 years
Max Lerner, Professor and columnist	Pulm metastes	D2	Buserelin chosen by patient.	Good Response Acid p'ase	80	Stained with Prost.	Mass in lung thought to be lymphoma	>5 years
George Sheehan, M.D., runner	Metastatic	D2	"	Seeks wisdom as death nears.	67	No grade	Fatigue	7 years
Susan Gilbert's husband, Prof. English	No	T3	Radical Prostatectomy	Death in the recovery room	60	Not given	Palpable nodule on routine physical	4 hours

TABLE 1

The range of time to death is huge. These men have lived from a few hours post-op (Gilbert) to more than ten years. Michael Korda is alive in 2012. This chart was shown at the Western Section of the A.U.A. in Las Vegas, NV, Nov. 2003.

narrative that would wither and erase the shadow of death."[386] This is a bit of French deconstruction[387] which did not work in a scientific sense, or any other sense. He died in a hurry. On the other hand, it did work metaphorically by allowing him to speak to us from beyond the grave via his book. It also appears that his doctors did a good job in their conventional job descriptions. Broyard could not sleep, urinate, or defecate upon presentation. His doctors fixed all those functions.

As the book opens, Broyard admitted that most professional writers live by secondary experience. He said, "I had been given a real deadline at last…I realized, for **the first time**, that I don't have forever." Later he wrote, "You expect that you are going to go on forever, that you're immortal."[388] This is a common phantasy among the humanists; they don't feel the biologic inevitability of death as M.D.s do.

Broyard's message is that we should savor every moment on this earth. He wrote, "When my wife made me a hamburger the other day, I thought it was the most fabulous hamburger in the history of the world."[389] As his male writer friends grouped around him after hearing the news, he felt a sense of superiority much as a mountaineer might who has returned from Everest missing his fingers. The mountaineer thinks to himself, "So what if they can still type; while they were typing, I was really living!"

His doctor's first estimate of his time on earth as "years" was wrong; he lived little more than one. That year was filled with talk. How he earned a living, he does not say. He was very grateful, for example, to the urologist who talked to him while looking up his urethra, a good lesson for all of us M.D.s. He explicitly points out, as does Korda, that status degradation, the toughest thing for a male primate, is the real pain of illness. Conversation restores status.

The loss of sex is the other. Broyard chose estrogen antagonism to male hormone as his way of fighting metastatic cancer after being offered surgical castration. The latter seemed to him to be death itself. He claims his erections were not interrupted by estrogen. This is possible since there is a famous paper in the Journal of Urology in the 1950s in which normal sex is claimed by about 20% of men castrated to control prostate cancer. Certainly, stallions, if trained to the artificial vagina prior to castration, will continue to mount after castration. I have heard a claim similar to Broyard's from a fifty-year-old patient at the Walla Walla V.A. whom I castrated to palliate an extensive, poorly differentiated carcinoma prior to the advent of Lupron and Zoladex. Broyard claimed that even if his erections failed in the future that he might continue to have a good sex life in his imagination. This is a bit narcissistic. What about his wife? This is, after all, the ultimate social act. Years before his own illness, Broyard described himself as moved to have intercourse with the head nurse at his father's cancer ward at King's County Hospital, and she with him. Sex is no small matter among literary artists.

Broyard, somehow, finds consolation in imagining that the cancer was caused by something he did in the past, an abnormal sex act in young adulthood. The thought that quantum mechanics reigns over DNA, that God rolls dice, is repellent to him. He feels he can live with personal guilt more easily than with a random universe. He wants to be alive when he dies. Maybe hammering himself with guilt is a way to do that.

He took an instant dislike to his first urologist whom he found to be too polite. He did not want his doctor "to be an amateur human being." He wants to know more about the prostate. He has no feeling for evolution nor has anybody ever told him that his prostate is the source of his libido. When it is full, as I see it, he feels like having intercourse. When it is empty, he does not. He wants his urologist to tell him things like that, but his urologist doesn't talk much.

He mistakes his unusually virulent cancer for all prostate cancers. At one point, he says that all prostate cancer victims will require a catheter. In this, he ignores the prevalence of the incidental, occult, autopsy cancers which cause urinary retention only very remotely in time, if at all. "Technical explanations flatten the story of illness." He is wrong here. Technical explanations *that are true* enrich it. For example, Broyard wrote, "What is my doctor thinking as he says, 'You have six to eighteen months.' I ask him about other patients, successes for his sake." He was worried about his doctor's mood if he failed constantly. To me, his doctor's statement was dramatic because it was true. In fact he lived fourteen months, as his wife wrote in her epilogue. It is only technical lies that are boring.

Broyard's call for dying to be "turned into some kind of celebration, a birthday to end all birthdays" is nonsense. The reason is that dying of cancer is an indistinct process. Parts of the patient, most importantly the brain, gradually change their function, well before the heart stops. The question is whose birthday party would it be? Patient X alert and well, or patient Y whose brain is affected by his cancer's occupation of his liver and by morphine?

He wants his friends to really know, through apt simile or metaphor, what his "illness is like" and, thereby, relieve his loneliness. His father, just before he died after months of pain from bladder cancer said, "I wish I had a hundred of my children here and their children."[390] I know this feeling. When I was suspended by my climbing rope upside down one hundred and thirty feet down in a dark crevasse on Mt. McKinley in 1967, my thought was that I was going somewhere my parents and siblings could not join me. I would be alone. Man is social and death is not social.

In regard to literary accounts of dying, Broyard cites the mountaineering literature in which those who have survived near fatal falls (like mine) do not experience anxiety but rather "a profound acceptance and an enhanced accelerated awareness and a greatly expanded sense of time." He is wrong about the acceptance. The mountaineering literature emphasizes that those *who survive* are rebellious regarding the outcome proposed by gravity. He is right about the expanded sense of time. This mountaineer's experience is very different from that of the cancer patients whose brain function is depressed by the parasitic cells hijacking his metabolism.

In his critical appraisal of the literature on death, Broyard cites Lisle Goodman's *Death and the Creative Life* most favorably. She found that what artists and scientists fear, is not death, but incompleteness. She therefore proposed, to Broyard's praise, "that we reckon our life backward, based on how much life we realistically estimate we have left to us." This is like the statement by the American Urological Association's committee on localized prostate cancer that advised, prior to initiation of treatment, consultation with actuarial life expectancy tables. As a 78-year-old white male, I have 9.3 years to live according to the Social Security actuarial tables. Ms. Goodman would have me celebrate this as my ninth birthday with a party. With the years left to me, I am going to seek immortality through artifacts *e.g.*, this book, as does another writer Broyard cites with favor, Ernest Becker's, *The Denial of Death*.

Cornelius Ryan's book, *A Private Battle*, assembled and authored by his wife Catherine Morgan Ryan after his death, is a better picture of an average cancer although, like Broyard's, Ryan's cancer is quicker to kill than average, significant prostate cancer. This thirty-year-old book is probably the best audit of United States urologists' performance in regard to this disease.

Ryan, author of *The Longest Day* and *A Bridge Too Far*, began to accumulate secret notes toward a book on his disease in July 24, 1970. It was in the form of more than 200 letters, 75 memoranda and medical reports, eight bulging notebooks, and six 120-minute tapes."[391] At the same time his wife and his secretary, both in secret and separate from each other, started files on his illness with the intent to publish. Why did the women do it? Catherine Ryan never says so explicitly, but it is clear she thinks her husband's illness and death are worth a report because Cornelius Ryan was not an amateur human being. He was a great human being. She convinces the reader that he lived his life abundantly, exhuberantly, and through primary experience according his private muse, not secondarily as Broyard did as a professional critic of the art of others.

The language of his needle biopsy report is out of date. Five cores are analyzed but they are not identified as to where in the prostate they came from. Ryan's biopsy says that all the cores were infiltrated with prostate cancer. That is an evil prognostic sign. The report also says, tellingly, that "one of the fragments contains a sympathetic ganglion and nerve and these are also extremely invaded by carcinoma." Since prostate cells have no business in the lymphatics tissue, this is evidence of metastatic disease in the perineural lymphatics. No Gleason grade regarding the degree of nuclear disorganization was given, nor was a widely published Mayo clinic grade of the time given, a major oversight by Memorial Sloan Kettering department of pathology.

Ryan began his dictation for his projected book on prostate cancer by acknowledging, at age 50, that he might be mortal. When this bubble burst, he felt lonely. His dictations were an attempt to feel less lonely. He says of the news he received the day before, "he means that I've got cancer." By now, the reader knows that 20% of men his age have prostate cancer and knows, therefore, that Ryan has almost no prognostic information so far except that he is symptomatic.

His first urologist is no consolation. The urologist wants to do a radical prostatectomy for cure. Cure to him is "to survive for 5 years following the surgery." Ryan found "...such a standard ludicrous." To him, "cure" was not the correct word to describe five years of survival. The reader, having read the previous chapters, should gag on the word too. His first urologist wanted to do the operation one week after making the diagnosis. This is too much hurry for Ryan. He is suspicious of the haste. He wanted to know how long he had had the disease. The reader knows, from the previous chapter, he has had it about 20 years. Ryan described symptoms of prostatitis of four months duration. Prostate cancer can cause prostatitis by blocking the ducts and entrapping ordinary bacteria that have swum up the urethra. His acute prostatitis caused urinary retention at 5:30 a.m., 4/18/70. This was treated with partial success with Negram, a well advertised drug at the time, but wrong because of a lack of penetration into the ducts. His symptoms of slow stream, burning and frequent urination did not improve. His local M.D., a generalist, not a urologist, then changed him to furadantin, again wrong for prostatitis, because it is active only in urine not the prostatic ducts. I did solo private practice in the same region three years later and used, with success, a powerful, broad-spectrum, semi-synthetic penicillin called carbenicillin when referred hard cases like Ryan.[392] Prostatitis has a reputation in urology for producing mental changes. It certainly did so in Ryan's case. He became totally unable to work on his last book, *A Bridge Too Far*.

I have come to see urinary frequency and incontinence in my forty years experience as an outsized threat to human males. This may be because during micturition we are vulnerable to attack by predators and rivals in romance. Twelve thousand years of life in cities is not enough time for evolution to select out apprehension during that act. It may even be that the inflamed prostate releases neuropeptides that modulate brain function just as leptin and gherlin from the stomach modulate brain function. Prostatitis patients sometimes seem crazy as jay birds. I have learned that they are not because they become normal when the bacteria are properly treated, as by carbenicillin, and then kept on a maintenance, suppressive therapy with trimethaprim. Even worse, Ryan stopped having intercourse with his wife because of the prostatitis. Periodic emptying of the gland would have been good for what ailed him, in a sense, the lancing of multiple tiny abscesses. This worried his wife since sex had been an important part of their marriage.[393] Ryan knew, via the insight into human nature afforded him by his experience as a journalist, of the unyielding importance of sex to women and suggested she find sex outside the marriage; he just did not want to be told about it.

His internist was not content with the urologists available in his region of Connecticut; he sent Ryan into New York City for a mere prostate biopsy. Ryan, like Broyard, discarded his first urologist; the urologist seemed to be in a big hurry to cut. He also sent out signals via his choice of words that even he did not believe in what he was recommending. Cognitive dissonance is hard to hide from an experienced interviewer. This first urologist wanted to do a radical prostatectomy. "It is the only cure, and I stress the word, that medical science knows today."[394] At that exact time, I was training in urology two miles away at the Presbyterian Hospital where the word "cure" was never used when referring to prostate cancer. Nor did the word ever appear in the Journal of Urology at that time. Ryan reports he said, "First, I don't know if there is a 'cure' for something like this, Doctor. You say so. Another doctor might not agree."[395] Ryan was concerned about the mental drive necessary to complete his next book. He worried (correctly in my view) about his motivation under the influence of female hormones or radical surgery. The doctor made no guarantees. He could not predict. He said, "I am sure you can adjust to the sex part of this. After all, you and your wife are surely not expecting any more children."[396] Surely this was the most jejune of his alleged comments and perhaps the one that caused him to lose Ryan as a patient. He also gave him fifteen years to live but only five years cancer free. Ryan, the literary-artist-journalist, gave himself three to three and a half years, an example of how an artist can resemble a scientist through close observation of nature.

He immediately saw, unlike Broyard, the implications for his earning power if knowledge of his diagnosis became generalized among editors; they would discard him. Publishers would cancel contracts. This is one of the reasons that prostate specific antigen (PSA) screening with its 70%-90% false positives can be so damaging. He worried about cost. We never learn whether or not he had medical insurance.

His first second opinion was from a fellow Irishman and urologist in New York. New York is an ethnic town in regard to medical care, not much melting in this particular pot. He tells Ryan that he can feel the cancer invading the seminal vesicle and that therefore radical surgery is not justified. He advised in 1970 exactly what we were taught to do at Presbyterian Hospital at the same time, systemic therapy, specifically suppression of male hormone. Ryan searched for experts to recommend other experts for another second opinion. Seven of twelve experts recommended Hugh Jewett of Johns Hopkins and Willet F. Whitmore, Jr. of Memorial Sloan-Kettering.

Dr. Whitmore's first recommendation, after looking at the slides, was to do nothing, surveillance for about five years, then hormones with a "hypothetical statistical fifteen years (of life) we are projecting here." Ryan quotes him as saying, "My approach over the last few years has been to veer away from prostatectomies. They produce greater surgical complications and mortality than the cancer itself…Now I am leaning toward a concept of studying the development of carcinoma cells." This is vague. He seems to have been talking about assessment of the individualized doubling times postulated by John Isaacs, Ph.D. in the previous chapter.[397] These doubling times were being reported for the first time in the 1970s. There is still no reference lab for such a determination in 2008, thirty years later. Dr. Whitmore then recommended a localized treatment, radioactive seeds for what he called in his notes "stage C," meaning he could feel the cancer out of the borders of the gland. But, the notes he gave Ryan's widow years later don't say "stage C." Whitmore is reported as saying he has patients doing well after 3-4 years with seeds but he also is reported as saying that is not nearly enough time to make a statement about prostate cancer. The old marker for prostate cancer in the bones, the acid phosphatase, was said to be normal. As Katherine Ryan recorded in a footnote, he never graded the cancer according to the Mayo Clinic standard published in 1922 but did note "perineural infiltration," *i.e.* metastases, in his note to the referring M.D. He then said in his consultation note, that if the tumor were to grow bigger locally, he would recommend either supervoltage radiation or his new project, I-125 seeds. Nowhere, is the intrinsically metastatic nature of the cancer overtly mentioned, but it is implied when he tells Ryan and his wife that his first intervention would be systemic anti-androgen therapy. Thus, in front of Ryan's journalist's gaze, he implicitly acknowledged that Ryan's cancer was systemic. Katherine Morgan Ryan correctly calls this "diffusion" of cancer cells in her footnote to this episode.

When they see Hugh Jewett of Johns Hopkins, he gives them a similarly mixed message: (1) the fact that all the needle biopsies were involved suggested disseminated disease and (2) the cancer formed glands; this meant it was close to its original cell type and therefore would be slow growing. He is then recommended yet another therapy, the supervoltage radiotherapy being done at Stanford, because of their ten-year statistics. The reader now knows from the previous chapter that (A) ten years is only a third of the time needed to draw a conclusion about prostate cancer. Ryan asked if he could get rid of the cancer forever. Jewett replies, "How would you like many years added to your life?" Of course, there was no data from localized therapy to support Jewett's offer then or now. My estimate of time gained by complete obliteration of the primary site based on the formula for compound interest and the known doubling time is 1.5 years added to life. In her account of the Jewett visit, Katherine Morgan Ryan seems to have been told that 15 years of follow up[398] is a minimum standard for a scientific report of the outcome of a localized intervention for prostate cancer, much as Whitmore implied. The reader also should know (B) that when the American Urological Association panel on localized prostate cancer reviewed Dr. Jewett's fifteen year evidence for radiation's effectiveness twenty-five years later, they found the evidence of insufficient quality to distinguish radiation from the natural history.

Six months after his first presentation and after seeing Dr. Jewett, Dr. Whitmore finally treated him with tetracycline, the first drug he received that was likely to be effective against prostatitis. This is a lesson for all urologists: pay attention to the chief complaint; do not forget it because you find an associated cancer.

Later, after the newly invented lymphangiogram ordered by Dr. Bagshaw in Stanford showed metastatic deposits in the lymph nodes, Dr. Bagshaw gave him three years, "…if you do nothing." Bagshaw opined that "…if the nodes were indeed malignant it meant that I (Ryan) had had cancer for more than two years." The reader now knows (C) that Ryan has had the cancer 18-35 years. In later notes written to his widow, Dr. Bagshaw claimed that many cancers can be "cured" even though they have spread to the lymph nodes. He does not give his definition of "cure." Is it five years without evidence of disease as per Ryan's first urologist? This is a strange definition of cure, not the one given in the glossary of this book. Dr. Bagshaw also wrote to Ryan's widow, "I am sure I did not know then how long the cancer had been present." That may be true. The subject of cancer cell kinetics is a gap in many physicians' education, particularly those from the far western United States, even though publications about cancer cell kinetics go back at least to fourteen years before the Bagshaw-Ryan meeting.[399] Twenty-four years after Ryan's death, the chairman and professor of Urology at Stanford withdrew his support for supervoltage radiation in a letter to the Journal of Urology.[400]

Dr. Whitmore recommended removal of Ryan's obviously cancerous lymph nodes as though that might have a curative effect. Speed was now said to be essential.[401] He recommended iodine seeds for the prostate. Nowhere was Ryan told the prevailing opinion in academic circles at the time, that this is an intrinsically metastatic disease.[402] Ryan asked, just before this operation, "If I'm sick, why don't I feel sick?" Apparently, Whitmore's tetracycline finally worked on his chronic prostatitis because earlier he said, "I've never felt better."[403] At the operation, all the iliac nodes were positive. His Irish friend, Dr. Nelligan, who referred him to Dr. Whitmore, said, "I hope it means he got them all." Everybody properly trained in cancer knew at that time and knows now that if cancer was grossly in those nodes, it was everywhere even though below the sensitivity threshold of Roetgen rays.

In regard to sex, Ryan's desire and performance became non-existent after the seeds were put in the prostate. His wife wrote, "My physical desires were unchanged even as Connie's were waning. It would have been easy to satisfy them (outside of marriage)."[404] She does not. However, her remarks point out that women in their late forties experience sexual desire as strongly as men at this age and that two people are being injured when this function is lost. These are two feisty characters and they clearly could have used the great peacemaker, the bone-hard penis, between them. Ryan experienced tremendous pain for 10 days after leaving the hospital, more pain than I would have thought from a large personal experience with that incision. The effect of the seed implant was to delay the systemic therapy, androgen ablation, he should have gotten early. One year after the cancer was first discovered, an intravenous pyelogram showed that one of his kidneys was completely blocked. He read in January 1972 that the mean time to death for a person with prostate cancer visible in the nodes is 5.5 years. That figure holds up today with notable exceptions on the long side. In April of 1972, his systemic disease was finally recognized from a radiolucent spot in the pelvic bones and by an elevation of his acid phosphatase level, what we used instead of PSA in those days. The lucent spot means that he had a poorly differentiated prostate cancer. He was at last put on 1 mg of Stilbesterol per day, a low non-clotting dose. This was two years too late, in my opinion. There was no excuse for the delayed prescription of anti-androgen therapy in Ryan's time except to allow time to collect money for the localized therapies. Urologists knew in the 1970s that anti-androgen therapy extended life. For example, Reed Nesbit wrote twenty years before Ryan's case in 1950 that "three and five year survival are significantly greater in endocrine-controlled patients than among others."[405] The Veterans Administration Cooperative Urological Research Group thought they could discern an advantage to early treatment through the noise of excess cardiovascular death caused by estrogen at 3 milligrams per day, three times the dose given Ryan, as early as 1967,[406] three years prior to the discovery of Ryan's cancer.

In February of 1973, Ryan experienced progressive skeletal pain. Dr. Whitmore switched him to a progestational drug. The switch did not work. He had to be admitted to Memorial Hospital in March of 1973 for intense pain. He had a high serum calcium level. This was caused by the cancer dissolving his bones and liberating the calcium into his blood stream. A high calcium level depresses both mental and cardiac function. One of his kidneys was blocked. Since his blood test for renal function showed insufficiency, he must have had extensive arteriosclerosis of the other in addition to cancer. A fifty-year-old man should have sufficient renal function after one kidney is taken out but Ryan was a smoker. At Memorial Sloan-Kettering he had a transurethral resection of the prostate. For the first time, we are told a grade on the pathology specimen, grade three out of a possible four, four being the worst case. He was started on two antimetabolic (chemotherapy) drugs. By May of 1973, he realized that the cancer was going to kill him. The chemotherapy cured the high blood calcium and should have been given far earlier in my opinion. Oncologists are doing so nowadays. There are better, safer cell poisons available. Constant bone pain told him he was alive. He writes a friend that he is "nearly broke. Medical costs have run close to $68,000…I've set up trust funds for the kids so they can get through college." There is no mention of life insurance or disability insurance. In July of 1973, Dr. Whitmore put him back on diethylstilbesterol 1 mg. He died of generalized metastases a little more than a year later in October of 1974, just after finishing *A Bridge Too Far*, a record of a campaign that mirrored Ryan's because it was ill conceived at the start by its specialist-generals except for Ryan's Irish urologist in the trenches of New York.

Michael Korda was the editor for *A Private Battle* but he does not seem to have learned from it. He, too, ended up at Johns Hopkins with a diagnosis of prostate cancer. There was a new chairman. The new chairman allegedly urged Mr. Korda to throw away the literature about radical prostatectomy he had obtained from a N.Y. radiotherapist because "everybody is different." If true, this was a statement that a science of medical care or science itself is impossible. It was in tune with the French deconstructionists that found a foothold in the United States at Johns Hopkins. The comment denied the possibility of medical wisdom through wide and long experience.

A strength of Korda's book is its description of the post operative period for the radical prostatectomy which Ryan, correctly in my view, turned down. We learn from Korda that the claim made by the enthusiasts for this operation, that the consequences of radical prostatectomy are negligible, is untrue. We learn from his interviews of others in a prostate cancer support group that man's ability to rationalize and justify his past decisions after the fact is infinite. Split brain humans will cook up preposterous explanations for what the opposite side of the brain has done.[407] We learn of a transient post-operative decrease in Korda's cognitive function, ability to maintain concentration, and ability to regulate his anger. It sounds to me like brain hypoxia caused by the period of low blood pressure and anemia he described in his post-operative period. Mountaineers who summit Everest without oxygen undergo similar changes. Members of my Mt. McKinley expedition were measured by a Ph.D. candidate to have had their word production per minute cut in half immediately upon our return to 10,000 feet from 20,000 feet. I was pretty drowsy myself until after two weeks at sea level. Hypoxic brain damage is a well-known complication of cardiac surgery[408,409] but it occurs after non-cardiac operations as well.[410] It can easily occur after radical prostatectomy if an age-related reduction in cardiac output is added to arteriosclerosis.

Korda discovered in his men's prostate cancer support group a persistent undercurrent of bitterness about having been deceived about the systemic character of this cancer from the get-go. The longest survivor was 15 years out, the figure mentioned by Dr. Whitmore to Ryan, but was on Strontium 89 for boney metastases. This patient's imminent death was on schedule for the 17.5 years ±1.8 years predicted by my paper in the British Journal of Urology. This man was post-radical prostatectomy, a fact not lost on the support group. The group knew through him that definitions of cure that refer to five and ten years are untrue. Both they and Korda appear unaware that the mean follow-up of the Johns Hopkins series was only four years at the time of Korda's procedure. After fifteen years follow-up, forty-one percent of this series had biochemical recurrence, a fact not mentioned in their many public relations newsletters. Korda's support group appears willing to draw inferences from hindsight that the new chairman at Johns Hopkins was not.

Max Lerner's account is the most profound and philosophic. His prostate cancer was diagnosed with a lung biopsy, something I saw reported in a journal for the first time in 2003.[411] He never interacted with institutionalized urology at all. He brought all of western literature to bear on the topic of man's mortality. Under the influence of medical neo-Luddites in California, he discovered, at the age of 80, the value of physical fitness and diet. The book worm became a gym rat. Threatened with orchiectomy, he found a pre-FDA approval protocol featuring Lupron that would save his testicles. In the eighth decade of an entirely intellectual life, he still valued his testicles highly on psychological grounds. He did not mention his sex life. He told us our job is to live intensely every day until we die, the same message as that of Thornton Wilder's *Our Town* as proclaimed by the late actor, Paul Newman.

George Sheehan, M.D., was an internist who, in his forties, gave up medical practice to run marathons, write, and speak on physical fitness. By scrupulous diet, furious exercise, and giving up smoking, he avoided an early cardiovascular death. This freed him to experience death later from prostate cancer. He chided himself for not having a yearly check-up despite the fact, that as an internist, he should have known that no study has demonstrated life extension from yearly check-ups. He had a naïve belief that early detection of cancer has produced measurable true cures, not spurious improvement caused by lead-time bias, for the common killers. His book on his prostate cancer, like Lerner's, is mostly about the aesthetics of time on earth well spent via scrutiny of the humanities. The most valuable medical content for the common reader is about importance of good pain control at the end by a pain specialist.

The last of my humanists, Susan Gilbert, was quoted in the chapter on complications of radical prostatectomy when she described her husband's postoperative death in the recovery room. Using her skill as a published poet, she makes us feel what she felt, a huge loss, a stone lodged permanently in her heart. The decision process that led to his operation was similar to that described by Ryan, and Korda.

A full professor of English consulted full professors of urology. In so doing, her husband did not distance himself from the culture which had given him tenure and a subsequent cozy life. Live by the sword, die by the sword. He did not realize he was caught up in an epidemic that afflicted his state, California, far more than the Northeast. If he had presented two years later, he probably would have escaped with his life as fashion changed. It seems possible that he, via his skill in the analysis of literature, could have spotted the rot in the narrative in favor of surgery just as Cornelius Ryan had gagged on a definition of cure as five years without disease. It was an English major that spotted the rot at Enron. But the professor of English was too trusting of the culture that had treated him so well. His red blood cells as a percent of his blood volume were reduced by 75%. His death appears to me to have been caused by diminished delivery of oxygen to his heart due to the reduced number of red cells to carry the oxygen mass and asymptomatic, coronary artery disease. The latter reduced his cardiac output but eluded standard pre-operative screens. He did not have the habits of exercise and diet discovered belatedly by Lerner when twenty years older. His death was a public event, like the break-up of the Challenger, an objective correlative to the 1% thirty-day death rate for radical prostatectomy published by Medicare for that year. The death of semi-retired Max Lerner in his eighties would have gone unremarked. The death in the recovery room of the chairman of English at a major University of California campus (Davis) had every ex-English major journalist in the central valley covering the story. Indeed, some of the motivation for this book comes from his widow's book, *Wrongful Death*. It raised the question of benificence, "Is one death too many for an operation that has not been proven to extend life?" Can humanists protect themselves when they find themselves in the medical-industrial complex? Is their literary education sufficient? It appears they are only partially defended. Ryan did not have a radical surgery. He was suspicious. But he did get radioactive seeds which delayed the systemic treatment (androgen ablation) that would have lengthened his life a little and may have hastened his death by causing dedifferentiation of his original middle grade cancer cells. Remember the radiolucent spots in his bones.

CHAPTER 14

The Instinct for Order: A Counter Reformation by the American Urological Association, the United States Congress, and the Veterans Administration.

"It was as if human society, having been torn apart, was starting to remake itself already, — as if with time there could have been kings and queens on that drifting hull, and maybe even priests." William Langeweshe's account of the last moments in the sinking of a ferryboat at night in a storm in the Baltic Sea. Atlantic Monthly, May 2004, p. 91.

About the time the European enlightenment was catching on in Scotland in the 1830s, David Hume said he did not know the proof for the belief that an experiment done yesterday would work equally well today. He saw no reason why the rules of the game in the universe might not change overnight. Let us recall that, in Hume's time, sixty-five thousand people still spoke Gaelic in Scotland, Ireland and Wales. Intellectual life was primitive on the edges of civilization. His position, when compared to beliefs in witchcraft unchanged from the time of Shakespeare, appeared rigorously modern. But in our time, we know many of the rules of the game of physics. We do not have to check the validity of Newton's gravity theorem prior to each spaceshuttle rocket launch. That time, we now know, is better spent checking O rings and the adhesion of foam insulation to the wings. We now know that, at the subatomic level, reality is statistical; dice are rolling. But we also know that the more quarks and mesons are aggregated, the more their behavior becomes predictable, lawful. Over-interpreters of Hume do not to admit that. They think that our impression of a connection between cause and effect may often be a function of our minds, not of events themselves.[412] They, like the chairman of Urology who saw Michael Korda, think that racks of books about the metastatic nature of prostate cancer in the past provide as a poor guide its probable future behavior in an individual. For super-Humeans, the contrary of a matter of fact is always possible.[413] Each person with prostate cancer is "a brave new world."

95

I am not keen on Hume, the philosopher. He does not smell of the lab. I like him better when he says that "...as an agent" he had no problem with the assumption that past behavior of nature was a practical guide to the future, *e.g.* the sun will rise tomorrow. We have two robots crawling about Mars because Newton was a reliable guide, not because of our fantasies. Similarly, we do not have to recheck the laws of biology as they apply to individuals every morning. But, it is crucial to acknowledge here that, compared to physics, chemistry, and geology, the application of the scientific method to medical care has happened 100 years later. The first controlled, prospective, randomized[414] trial of a medical therapy in people occurred in my lifetime, in the 1948 trial of streptomycin.[415] My grandfather and his colleagues at the Cornell Medical School in the 1920s and 1930s were flying blind in their attempts at scientific therapeutics.

Even after the clarity introduced by the streptomycin trial, controlled, randomized, prospective trials in therapeutics are rarely funded. If funded, they are terminated prior to sufficient accrual. For example, the first randomized, controlled, and prospective study of radical prostatectomy and of androgen deprivation in the history of the world lost its funding by Congress before it had accrued significant numbers. It was run by the Veterans Administration Cooperative Urological Research Group from 1967 to 1975. We call it the VACURG study. At 10 years, the small size of the group permitted a 66% chance of overlooking a 50% improvement.[416] At 23 years, this study showed no difference, when corrected for an age imbalance, between those who had undergone radical prostatectomy and controls in regard to death, all causes.[417] Nobody cared. There were only 39 patients in the non-operated, control group and 37 in the operated group. Compare these numbers to the 400 patients randomized in 1989 by a Scandinavian group and the 2000 persons planned for the Veterans Administration revival of this same research problem called the PIVOT trial. The cancellation of VACURG was penny wise and pound foolish. Congress, at the time, was spending millions for veterans' prostate cancer and was beginning to spend billions for older Americans under Medicare/Medicaid.

A decade after the VACURG study, and two years before the peak of the epidemic of care, the increasing rate of prostate biopsy which started in 1985, and the subsequent jump in radical prostatectomy numbers provoked a series of papers. One came from the University of Chicago, a bulwark for science in this topic because of the Nobelist, Charles Huggins. It showed that surveillance followed by androgen ablation for signs of progression had results equal to surgery. Because of the University of Chicago paper and others like it, the American Urological Association convened the Prostate Cancer Clinical Guidelines Panel in 1989, to conduct a comprehensive survey and meta-analysis of published data.[418] They finished their report six years later, in 1995, three years after the peak of the epidemic of radical surgery.

The 1995 report said the following: "All the studies finally selected by the panel provided useful information, but most were case series not subjected to the rigors of a carefully performed, *prospective, centrally controlled* clinical trial... Because of the particular attributes of this disease, such as *high histologic prevalence*, yet variable natural history, treatment outcomes data from *uncontrolled* trials can be even less reliable than usual…Many articles do not report all outcomes (such as cancer specific survival, metastasis-free survival and tumor free survival). .. There are also few data on high-grade tumors managed by surveillance…Many articles do not specify the ages of the patient…many articles reporting complications from treatment do not report zero complications…A common problem with prostate cancer series… is the reporting of endocrine therapy for patients developing recurrence after surgery or radiotherapy. The timing of administration may not be clearly detailed …(There is) Publication bias:…studies with negative or equivocal results are less likely to be submitted for publication and less likely to be published…The data available do not always reflect the many changes in treatment modalities that have occurred over the past two decades."[419]

Even then, back in 1995, the panel said, "PSA is not prostate cancer specific…it lacks sufficient sensitivity and specificity to be the ideal screening test for prostate cancer." Moreover, they pointed out that a major problem with using low PSA levels as a sign of successful treatment is that "androgen-insensitive cells do not produce and secrete PSA to the same degree as androgen-sensitive cells. Thus, patients with progressive disease after androgen deprivation therapy may in fact have a low or stable serum PSA concentration." This is seven years before I wrote my chapter on PSA. So my chapter is not an outlaw statement. It is inside the groupthink of my specialty.

The panel went astray when it stated that "androgen deprivation therapy remains a palliative treatment for most patients" when in fact, at the time, we knew, by comparing cancer specific survival in the pre- and post-endocrine eras, that patients were living longer. We knew, in the rat, that there was a 42% gain in longevity, early versus late.[420] The panel correctly said, "in particular, randomized, controlled trials are needed to compare surveillance with accepted active treatments.[421]…The fifteen year progression data are sparse, variable, and uncertain."[422] Thus, they appeared to have been aware that follow-up to >15 years, as per my publication in the British Journal of Urology, was necessary. The panel concluded that it would therefore be methodologically unsound to compare treatment modalities directly with regard to survival and progression.[423]

The panel did quote under the heading "Basis for Management by Surveillance" a prostate cancer prevalence of 80% in older men[424] (9% is the prevalence in forty year olds).[425] But they defined cure as "lifetime freedom from disease."[426] This is not the plain meaning of the word, cure. The plain meaning of cure is that the cancer will never get you no matter how long you live. By the American Urological Association definition, an automobile accident or a heart attack could cure a patient in his tenth postoperative year even though, without the accident or heart attack, he would die of prostate cancer about his 17th year post-discovery. An auto accident would satisfy the panel's "lifetime freedom from disease" definition. It even allows Cornelius Ryan's first urologist's five year definition. Remember Ryan found it ridiculous. By this definition, Professor Gilbert was cured when he died in the recovery room five hours after his prostatectomy. He appeared free of prostate cancer for his lifetime. Unless we are going to give into French deconstruction's reign of terror declaration that words have no fixed meaning, diction matters. The A.U.A. panel's definition of cure is not the plain meaning. It does not pass muster.

The panel defined the word, option, better. It is a term of art in medical policy formation derived from Eddy.[427] The panel said it was a choice made when "the health…outcomes of the interventions are not sufficiently well known to permit meaningful decisions."[428] I have always taken the panel's word, meaningful, to mean scientific, rational, or informed. My problem with the word meaningful is that all decisions are meaningful. Poor decisions may mean the decision maker is ignorant, demented, psychotic, or culture bound.

The A.U.A. panel used the word, option, to define their policy regarding radical prostatectomy, radiotherapy, and surveillance. By giving all three modalities the same word as a rating, option, they said that each modality had an equal claim on the attention of our citizens.[429] They said that the published results made surgery and radiation equavalent as a choice to no treatment plus an assumed but unstated androgen deprivation treatment at some point. This is the only policy statement I know by a surgical society which states that a cancer operation with intent to cure in their specialty is equivalent to doing nothing. The prose of the A.U.A. statement is tortured. I have used the portability of equivalence, an axiom from Euclid, to tease this meaning out of the 1995 white paper. Here is Euclid. If A =B and C=B, then A=C.

When the American Urological Association (A.U.A.) rewrote this policy statement for the public in a glossy brochure, they did not disclose to the public the meaning of the Eddy derived word, option. Never one to lie low, I protested this omission in the brochure with a letter to the A.U.A. in 1998. I received back a letter from an officer, Martin Resnick, M.D., which clearly stated that the panel regarded the outcome of surveillance, i.e. the natural history or no treatment, to be equal to the outcomes of radical surgery and radiation.[430] In spite of Martin Resnick's reply to me, the A.U.A. brochure was not revised to reveal that the word, option, is a term of art. It is grimly ironic that Dr. Resnick wrote an editorial nine years later in 2007 about the difficulty he had in choosing the option of bone marrow transplant for his recently diagnosed leukemia. He had not come to grips with the fact that when a cancer specialist, in this case his oncologist, uses the word, option, he has run out of science and is engaged in commerce. Dr. Resnick died six months after his editorial. Apparently his oncologist did not have a science based remedy. The bone marrow transplant may have killed him.

Because of the cost of the epidemic to Medicare, the United States Congress's Office of Technology Assessment (OTA), since disbanded in a foolish economy move, dove into these muddy waters in 1995, six months earlier than the A.U.A, with a publication called "Costs and effectiveness of prostate cancer screening in elderly men."[431] They concluded that "research has not yet been completed to determine whether systemic, early screening for prostate cancer extends lives." They noted the wide prevalence of asymptomatic occult prostate cancers with advancing age. In a footnote, they told us that the U.S. Agency for Health Care Policy and Research (AHCPR) had not issued any guidelines concerning prostate cancer screening with PSA.

The O.T.A. alluded to private sector A.U.A. and the American Cancer Society policies which were in favor of screening at that time. On the other hand, the American College of Pathology was quoted as not recommending PSA screening among the general asymptomatic population,[432] and as saying that "the level at which a PSA measurement should be considered suspicious is controversial."[433] The O.T.A. went on to say that the transrectal ultrasound image was not specific for cancer but useful in directing biopsies. They said, "No trial showing which of the various treatment strategies saves the most lives (if any) has yet been completed." The O.T.A. predicted 20 persons per 100,000 screenings were predicted to die from biopsy or treatment complications.[434] This is not far from my estimates in the earlier chapters on complications. The O.T.A. pointed out that researchers were just starting randomized trials of adequate power as of 1995, but that 10-15 years would be required to accrue sufficient patient cancer deaths. In their view, Medicare coverage of PSA screening would lead to an uncertain health benefit. The O.T.A. was disbanded in an economy move by the Congress, just as the V.C.U.R.G. prospective, randomized, controlled study of radical prostatectomy of the 1960s was disbanded years earlier. These cancellations have cost us taxpayers millions.

I conclude from the A.U.A. and O.T.A. reports that disinterested, government observers did not find a basis in science for the epidemic of diagnosis, surgery, and radiation that peaked in 1992. Because of that gap, two prospective randomized studies were begun in 1995. One of them, a Veterans Administration study called PIVOT, was and remains confounded by the fact that androgen ablation can be done at any time. This is the same critique I have made of the Swedish study.[435] Androgen ablation would occur early in the radical surgery cohort because in the 30% to 60% of operations, cancer is found at the margins, just as in Young's five patients in 1910. The surveillance group would get androgen ablation later because there is no pathology specimen to ring the alarm of long-standing systemic disease. We know from an animal study and several clinical series that early androgen is better than late. For that reason, predictably the surgery group would do better. As the results came out in recent years, I was surprised to see that the surgery group did not do statistically better; this negative result is part of the crux of this book's argument.

We know that only one out of 380 persons over 50 who have prostate cancer dies of it. Thomas Stamey, retired professor and chairman of Urology at Stanford, compared autopsy data of prevalence to cancer specific death rates and came up with this ratio in 1983. With such a low frequency of deaths relative to the prevalence of histologic cancers at autopsy, I calculate that a series of 249,035 persons is required to detect a >10% improvement.[436] A 10% improvement was sought by Swedish-Holmberg series cited above. You would need an equal number of controls. *This means, to achieve statistical significance, a half million men would have to be followed for thirty years.* Such a study is not practical in our commercial society nor even in socialist countries like Sweden and England. The current Veterans Administration PIVOT study, as stated earlier, only envisions 2,000, not 200,000, entrants to each wing. But accrual has stopped at 700 in the PIVOT series in our version of socialized medicine, the V.A. system. The V.A. is 10% of medical care in the United States. If the proposition that radical surgery and radiation lengthen cancer specific life cannot be proven under our version of socialism, I see no chance that it can be proven in our anarchic private sector.

When Kenneth Kizer, M.D., was the director, the Veterans Administration system adopted a scientific attitude. Kizer had led the charge to convert the V.A.'s surgery from inpatient to outpatient. He took the resultant savings and bought thousands of personal computers and commissioned software written for a paperless, computerized, M.D.'s chart. The socialist V.A. was and remains ten years ahead of the private sector in this area. It is of general interest, therefore, to ask how this progressive, capitated, government-sponsored, evidence-based HMO responded to the epidemic of prostate cancer diagnosis and therapy occurring all around it in the 1980s and 1990s.

At the Fresno, California, V.A. Medical Center where I worked starting in 1994, radical prostatectomies doubled from an average of 10 per year in the 1980s to 20 in 1991, whereas Medicare in the nation at large sextupled its total. This V.A. abruptly changed course in 1994, the year of my arrival, and only did one radical prostatectomy in 1995.[437] For patients aged over seventy-five, the downturn in biopsies began in 1990 in my facility, whereas the decline in biopsies started three years later, 1993, for Medicare at large.

The director of the entire system, K. Kizer, M.D., came out against using the PSA test for prostate cancer without a prior counseling session with the vet about the risks and rewards. He noted that there had been no demonstration of life extension by the therapies offered after screening. As a result of his opposition, the V.A. system as a whole did not buy into the epidemic of 1987 to 1995. Prostate cancer was a cost, not a profit, center in this island of socialism. For example, the number of V.A. radical prostatectomies nationwide increased less than twofold from 1986 to 1996[438] instead of the six-to-seven-fold increase seen in the quasi-free market Medicare system. The V.A. system even got the message about not operating on persons older than seventy-five in 1991, a year earlier than fee-for-service Medicare. It did one such operation in 1995. In the age 65-75 group, the V.A. system lost its enthusiasm in 1993, a year later than the Medicare system. In the same age group, the West North Central V.A. rate dropped in half from 1993 to 1995. By contrast, the age 55 to 64 group started to go up in 1988, the year after PSA was introduced, and has kept on rising steadily to more than double its former rate, as has the age 45 to 54 group.

The geographic variations in regard to operating on those older than seventy-five were similar to Medicare. There was a sevenfold difference between low-use areas (East, South Central) and high-use areas (North Central). The map of frequencies of all ages (aggregated) looks different than the Medicare map; it shows a strong band of high-frequency states running down the center of the country with an outlying peak in the

West North Central district. Some western states that are high frequency on the Medicare map are low on the V.A. map, *e.g.* Wyoming, Nevada, Montana, the Dakotas, Kansas and Texas. Thus, a socialist system led by an M.D. with a commitment to science participated reluctantly in the epidemic. Alas, the nail that sticks up higher than the others will be hammered down in any large bureaucracy and so Dr. Kizer left the system, a hero to some of us.

CHAPTER 15

Deconstruction and the Great Disruption.

"In the baseball of the future the players and fans will mingle as equals on the field..."—Garrison Keillor

About the time that radical prostatectomy and radiation utilization peaked, the murder rate in cities over one million peaked in 1992; car thefts in Fresno, California and suicides age 15 to 24 years nationally peaked in 1994.[439] Why these correlations? I think Francis Fukuyama's concept of "the great disruption," a period of social disorder which he says peaked in 1992, explains the coincidence.

A baleful predictor of the coming wave of disorder was a conference in 1986 at Johns Hopkins, that sought to legitimize in the United States the writings of two Frenchman, Michael Foucault and Jacques Derrida. They said, at their most extreme, that because science is recorded in words and because words have no fixed meaning, science is a social construct, an attempt by Northwest Europeans to hang on to power. It has no intrinsic validity. They ordered a roll-back of The Enlightenment. For a devastating characterization of this line of thought, here is Professor Steven Pinker in his recent best seller on human nature thus:

"This whole enterprise is based on an unstated theory of human concept formation: that conceptual categories bear no systemic relation to things in the world but are socially constructed (and therefore can be reconstructed)...Yes, every snowflake is unique, and no category will do complete justice to every one of its members...but intelligence depends on lumping things that share properties, so that we are not flabbergasted by every new thing we encounter...This kind of inference works because the world really does contain ducks, which really do share properties. If we lived in a world in which walking, quacking objects were no more likely to contain meat than did any other object, the category 'duck' would be useless and we probably would not have evolved the ability to form it."[440]

Prof. Pinker goes on with rapier thrusts but, to cut the story short, I prefer an ad hominem attack. The man who first brought deconstruction to America, a Yale professor, Paul de Mann, wrote propaganda for the Nazis during World War II. It was the Nazis who exploited the power of mass communication (via radio) for evil. For them, words had no fixed meaning and lies repeated often enough became true.

I, following the trail of Prof. Pinker and Prof. Lehman, believe this set of ideas to be hogwash, but not to be dismissed easily. Their siren call has been answered by quite a few men of goodwill and political weight. They have drunk the cool-aid.[441] For example, the benign prostatic hypertrophy (BPH) described in this book was declared in 1996 by an anthropologist in a professional venue to be a social construction.[442] This is folly. The six patients with 150 to 250 grams of BPH I resected in the Veterans Administration system and then reported to the Western Section of the American Urological Association were not figments of a febrile imagination. When magnified by the lens of the cystoscope, they looked to be immense collections of muons, quarks, and mesons that fully justified operating sessions of one-and-a-half hours, repeated a week later in the case of the 250 gram tumors. Similarly, there are facts about prostate cancer *e.g.*, the 3.6% of men who die of it, that are true. They are not social constructs. But if you think Jacques Derrida and Michael Foucault are too esoteric to have penetrated into departments of Urology, think again. I had a conversation in 2000 with a professor and chairman of Urology in a respected state university who said, in regard to the prostate cancer debates, that it was all just words with no fixed meaning, that therefore the truth was indeterminate. This happened. My wife heard it.

Here is an example of the penetration of French deconstruction, this time inside United States urology: about 1995, I volunteered to give a lecture to the non-M.D. support staff in our clinic about the therapy of erectile impotence, which I had ramped up upon my arrival. I told them that a famous paper in the early 1950s in the Journal of Urology had reported that almost a quarter of men in their fifties castrated for prostate cancer continued to have erections and a sex life. An R.N. assigned to oncology in attendance told me, by telling them that fact, I was being "patriarchal." I was speechless at the time because I had not yet studied this new intellectual fashion. I could not interpret the semiotics even though English was her first language but now I know. It goes like this. Because I told her something she did not already know, I was engaging in a power play to set up a hierarchy with me, a male and an M.D. at the top. She apparently would rather have not known what I was telling her. This would preserve the egalitarianism that she and the French deconstructionists cherish. I am not saying that I ever heard the name of Derrida mentioned at this institution. I am saying I believe that French nihilism disguised as sophisticated thought had filtered down from the parent university to this satellite, training facility and thence into R.N. education. The R.N. above seemed to think I was engaging in propaganda.

Francis Fukuyama picked up the theme of science as propaganda. He wrote:

"A society built around information tends to produce more of the two things people value most in modern democracy—-freedom and equality. Freedom of choice has exploded, in everything from cable channels to low cost shopping outlets to friends met on the Internet. Hierarchies of all sorts, political and corporate, have come under pressure and begun to crumble...Marriages and births declined and divorce soared; one out of three children in the United States and more than half of all children in Scandinavia were born out of wedlock...trust and confidence in institutions went into a forty year decline."[443]

I cannot quarrel with him. The wife of one of the Veterans Administration psychologists was murdered in her home during a robbery in Fresno in 1994, the year we moved there; it was a war zone. I believe a parallel attrition of social capital (Fukuyama's term) occurred in urology, starting in 1983. It became disorderly. A sign was the high rate of margins positive for cancer in the radical prostatectomy specimens sent from the operating room to pathology, even in the best university settings. The margin positive rate ranged from 30% to 60%. This meant that within a week of the surgery, nobody could maintain the fiction that surgery done for cure had cured in the plain meaning of the word. They were not suffering pre-op except mildly from BPH and so could not be called patients. But now they were patients, sufferers. I believe that in the 1960s and 1970s, the Department of Pathology at Columbia Presbyterian would have called the question by communicating with members of the Department of Internal Medicine that the Department of Urology had run amok. The internists would have stopped referring to any urologist who produced such specimens. In fact, I remember a young attending urologist at that hospital in 1973 showing me a conventional x-ray film of vertebrae spotted with prostate cancer. He had done a radical prostatectomy only six months before. He told me that he would stop doing the operation; it was nonsense. He urged me, as chief resident, to eschew it just as Robert Lich, M.D., at his retirement as chairman of Urology at Louisville, had urged his successor in 1974 to avoid it.[444] I did avoid the operation. No more radical prostatectomies were performed at the V.A. in Huntingtion, West Virginia, after I moved there in 1983.

How could this amount of cognitive dissonance flourish? One reason was that, as another result of the anti-hierarchical spirit of the times, urologists and radiation oncologists no longer chose the therapy for the citizens. In tune with the egalitarian goals of French deconstruction, what I call reign of terror democracy, the citizens had become empowered. They were freed from premedical courses in college, four years of graduate study for the M.D. degree and six years of on the job experience previously thought necessary to make grave medical decisions of this sort. Our men were now to be given a menu featuring their options, that loaded word. In this brave new world, the M.D. was a mere waiter in a classy restaurant with a menu rather than an authority on disease and therapeutics.

I experienced this development first hand when I moved from the Walla Walla V.A. to the Minneapolis V.A. in 1993. One of the first patients assigned to my clinic told me he had made up his mind and that he was choosing radical prostatectomy from his list of options. This was the year after the peak of the epidemic of radical surgery from which I had been largely isolated. Walla Walla, Washington, is an elegant, three college town with the look and feel of New England. Some of the Victorian houses have upstairs ballrooms. Again, as when the R.N. mentioned above called me "patriarchal," I was rendered speechless. I had become accustomed to the hierarchy between me and the veterans in which ten years of education after college meant something. I had actually attended a small Catholic hospital in Manhattan, St. Elizabeth's, in the 1970s where, when I entered the nurses station as a young graduate urologist with no seniority except my M.D. and residency certificate, all the nurses stood up at attention and awaited what I had to say. By the late 1980s, when I came into a nurses' station in Minneapolis, I was totally ignored. I was not used to this new social order. I told the patient that I too had made a decision. I would refer him to another M.D. on staff at the V.A.

Of course, at no time during these years would an M.D. present a patient with pneumonia a menu of antibiotic options and ask the sufferer which medicine he wished. It was unique to the cancers in which scientists had no saleable cures that the hierarchy between M.D. and sufferer was opportunistically extinguished.

The antidote to the false vision of equality skewered by Garrison Keillor in the quotation above is, in my opinion, for the M.D. to spend time in a laboratory with the animals both in medical school and residency training. It is there that the M.D. gains the confidence to say that the biologic facts are what they are, not what the herd is muttering for commercial gain. I did this on three separate occasions totaling almost two years as a medical student and urology resident. Working with the animals, as distinct from a patient care setting, you have sufficient control so that you are able to sense the laws of nature that exist with or without a man to observe them. It is what Walt Whitman meant when he wrote, "Oh vast rondure spinning in space." A chilly, lonely vision. But there it is.

What the M.D. researcher comes up with after glimpsing, feeling with his fingers, the autonomy of nature is unlikely to be propaganda. He becomes expert in his topic no matter how much the French deconstructionists (and the Quakers!) hate hierarchy. A robust understanding of mammalian chemistry and structure gained in the lab doing original work sustains the M.D. in the seriously conflicted clinical scene where leveling social and political forces have real power.

To fight French deconstruction the M.D. must write, speak, and publish his/her thoughts, case reports, and clinical tricks. I started to do this at age forty, and found out that it was not difficult to publish a letter or have an abstract accepted in a regional meeting if I approached my subject as an expert. It is by writing and standing on his hind legs at the podium that the M.D. solidifies his thoughts to the point they are unassailable even though unpopular. Samuel Johnson said, "It focuses a man's mind wonderfully to know he is going to be hanged in a fortnight." By committing himself in public to positions in medical care, any M.D., not just full-timers in the universities, can prove that science is more than a record of who is on top of whom in a hierarchy.

CHAPTER 16

Why Didn't the Universities Stop the Epidemic?

In alio peduclum vides, in te ricinum non vides —Petronius[445]

In the university hospitals, as per Emerson's dictum, "things are in the saddle and ride mankind." Faculty practice plans pay more to those who admit more to the university hospitals and do procedures than to those who admit less and do fewer procedures. The directors of the hospital and associated clinics are paid well into six figures. At the university of Pittsburgh hospital system, they are paid more than that according to the Wall Street Journal. Professors of surgery and radiation oncology who are supposed to be living on money from an endowment are only partially supported in their lifestyle. They earn as much or more from fees for service in the faculty practice plan than they are paid in salaries. The profits after that go back to the dean's office where they are used to pay pediatricians and general practitioners. Gone is the spirit of the period 1910-1965 when department chairmen, interested only in research and teaching, were content with a fixed income from bonds.

This spirit dates from the report in 1910 by Abraham Flexner, a successful prep-school headmaster from Kentucky, at the behest of the Carnegie Foundation. He wrote a report that closed two thirds of the medical schools in the United States. The report said that most of them were commercial, proprietary operations undeserving of the public's confidence in their product. Elizabeth Blackwell, the first woman physician educated in the United States, went to such a school. So did Flexner's brother who went on to found the Rockefeller Institute. The schools on his hit list were then bankrupted because the state medical boards would no longer give licenses to M.D.s whose degrees originated from them. Potential students did not want to pay them tuition. After Flexner moved to a Rockefeller sponsored 'think tank' on education, it gave massive endowments to medical schools he favored to foster the transition to salaried, full-time chairmen of medicine, surgery, and Ob/Gyn. They clipped coupons from bonds instead of sending out monthly bills. They were supposed to teach and discover what was good for the body rather than what was good for their pocketbook.

Early recipients were such private schools as Johns Hopkins, Yale, the University of Chicago, Washington University in St. Louis, my alma mater, Columbia's College of Physicians and Surgeons, and then surprisingly, a state supported school, the University of Iowa. They all complied at first when offered sufficient money. Harvard came in late, loudly protesting about the loss of private practice income.

Johns Hopkins, Washington University in St. Louis, and Iowa, early recipients of Rockefeller money, have all been prominent in the prostate cancer literature, but not always for the better, in my opinion. Flexner wanted the medical schools out of commerce. He also required them to have access to hospitalized patients via the appointment of the university professors as chiefs of service in hospital departments. This was easy to arrange at Johns Hopkins Medical School because it owned its own hospital as a result of its founding bequest. Hospital ownership looked like an advantage in the late nineteenth century when hospital deficits were covered by philanthropy. When I was a medical student, 1961-1965, the wards of Columbia Presbyterian Hospital in New York City contained a scattering of middle class persons who could actually pay a small charge and whose conditions were deemed interesting by the medical or surgical chief resident. The destitute were referred to a local public hospital. But this paradigm changed drastically with the Medicare/Medicaid legislation of 1965, the year I graduated from medical school.

The thesis of this chapter is that this legislation unraveled Flexner's reforms. The university affiliated hospital where I did my internship sent a representative to Washington D.C. to find out what it would mean for this particular hospital. I overheard a conversation about his report when he came back. He was said to have said, "They are loading a train with gold and it is headed our way." What I saw immediately as an intern with a short white jacket, was that the chief resident in surgery, who had previously labored in obscurity in the charity clinic in a short white jacket similar to mine, began to wear the long white coat of a fully trained surgeon in a newly constructed private practice office suite. The hospital then billed the federal government and the state of New York on his behalf and that of his supervisors for services previously provided for free.

Money poured into what were called faculty practice plans. The chairman and professors, whose real income from the interest on the bonds that backed their endowed professorships had shrunk because of the cruel Johnsonian inflation, began to outstrip inflation with clinical fees laundered by passage through the dean's office. In the upper Midwest, a professor and chairman of Urology was reported by the Wall Street Journal to have taken home about about $400,000 in 1998 ($1,539,032 in 2018 corrected for inflation) at a time when the average urologist in private practice paid taxes on half of that. What was left over after agreed upon, contractual limits went from the faculty practice plan to the dean's office where he took 10% for the school in a typical arrangement. The dean used the remainder to run the medical school and pay attractive salaries to low earners. Income from commercial, fee-for-service faculty practice plans constitutes about 80% of medical school revenues currently. About 70% of that figure comes from Medicare /Medicaid.

These enormous flows of new money caused a rise in the number of faculty members in the clinical disciplines, who earned a median salary of $160,000,[446] and a corresponding decrease in the number of basic science faculty members[447] whose median salary was $78,000. It would be the latter who would do the animal experiments that form the foundation of clinical practice according to Flexner's model. Business school techniques achieved prominence among M.D.s running medical schools.

The party lasted eighteen years. Then two things happened within Medicare: (1) reimbursement to M.D.s changed from the lunatic "usual and customary" sliding fee scale passed by Congress in 1965 to a fee schedule. This was price fixing. This brought down, for example, the effective payment for a radical prostatectomy down from about $2500 in the 1970s to about $1200 currently. Corrected for inflation that is about $400 1976 dollars. For a transurethral resection of the prostate (TURP) I get about 1/6 the buying power (considering inflation and the fee schedule reductions) compared to what I received in private practice in New York City in 1976. (2) Hospitals got a fee schedule also called "diagnostic related groups" in 1983. This was price fixing again. They were paid by diagnosis whether the diagnosis had deeper issues or not. By 1986, hospital executives said profits had decreased 47.1% since 1985.

Immigration restrictions against foreign medical graduates, in place since the 1920s, were also relaxed in 1965. The doubling of United States graduates between 1965 and 1980, plus the flood of foreign medical graduates, created the first real competition in American medicine since Flexner's 1910 revolution. In 1983, the year of the revival of the radical prostatectomy and the start of the diagnostic related groups, Congress provided extra payments to teaching hospitals to cover special costs associated with medical education. These graduate education payments increased with the number of trainees, and hospitals responded by increasing the number of interns and residents.[448] The number of graduates of foreign medical schools in United States residencies increased from 10,000 to 20,000 per year.[449] This has changed the ratio of United States graduates to foreign medical graduates in practice from one in six in 1985 to one in three in 2002 since the foreign medical graduates almost never go home. The United States outsourced medical education to foreign lands. It is no longer easy for a United States graduate M.D., even from a 'Flexner' university, to earn a living.

Since about 1990, the advent of managed-care insurance schemes, Flexner's university hospitals, over-staffed with salaried medical school personnel from the easy money days, have been in permanent crisis. Life has been quite different from the cozy 1930s when the full-timer's bonds appreciated in value due to deflation. My urologic training facility, Columbia Presbyterian Hospital, avoided bankruptcy caused by managed care by merging with New York Hospital, an affiliation of Cornell Medical School and a long time rival. The fusion was successful in the sense that John D. Rockefeller's "ruinous competition" was avoided. Market share gave them monopoly power and they could bargain with managed care insurance schemes that rapidly colluded to form monopolies themselves. I see advertisements for patients in the Sunday New York Times magazine section every Sunday, *e.g.* the Mt. Sinai Hospital in New York paid for a full page advertisement in June 2007 which said that their new radical prostatectomy surgeon seldom had erectile impotence as a complication of his work. I see billboards in Westchester County advertising what was formerly called the Columbia Presbyterian Medical Center. I also see their associated College of Physicians and Surgeons edging away from the Flexner mandated hospital connection and toward its university sponsor through a name change of its health science schools. An attempted merger between the private Stanford University Hospital, and the state of California hospital owned University of California at San Francisco about the same time was catastrophic and undone within two years. It seemed to me, from my salaried, full-time, 'fox-hole' in the Veterans Administration from 1986 to 2002, that my colleagues in academia and in private practice were pre-occupied with staying alive economically.[450] The application of scientific principles to prostate cancer was an after thought in desperate times.

Medicare legislation directed at the hospital component created trouble at a deeper level. It mandated a management technique devised by Alexander Demming for the manufacture of automobiles. Demming sought a uniformity of process which would guarantee uniformity of output. This elevated process over outcome. It was successful because of the uniformity of input in his business. Medical care does not have that uniformity of input. It has the opposite. Consider the following quote from Brook *et al* in the New England Journal of Medicine about three invasive procedures where abusive over-utilization seemed to be occurring. "...Our findings about the relation between the volume of the procedures and the appropriateness further confirm the need to measure the appropriateness of care directly. *How well a procedure is performed is not a proxy for whether it needs to be performed.* ...If we do nothing to assess appropriateness (the university function), we could end by developing policies that improve the level of quality at which a procedure is performed but lower the population based measures of health, because the wrong people are receiving the procedure, and thus the net health risk exceeds the benefit."[451]

Medicare was an economic vector that caused the universities to fall asleep at the switch.' But there were political vectors as well. For example, as a result of egalitarian forces re-activated by the civil rights revolution for African Americans in the United States, the pool of women applicants increased from 20% in 1974 to 45% in 1999. The percentage of men dropped from 80% to 55%. While there are obvious advantages to giving women equal access to medical training, from the point of view of medical research, there is a drawback. Women recruited into hard science tend to drop out in far larger numbers than men. Lawrence Summers, when president of Harvard, lost his job by noting this fact and suggesting that it might be related to differences in brain function. In medical life, women tend to go into the more social specialties such as family practice and psychiatry. I know of one female urologist who, appalled by the morbidity of radical prostatectomy, retrained into psychiatry. The non-surgical specialties do not typically require protected time at the laboratory bench away from patients as do the surgical disciplines.

Since the Nuremburg war crimes trials after World War II, the civilized West has required of itself animal experimentation by presumably Flexner's endowed full-timer prior to human experimentation.[452] The code says, "The experiment should be so…based on the results of animal experimentation…that the anticipated results will justify the performance of the experiment."[453] This minimal requirement of post-World War II society for preliminary animal experimentation has never been met in the case of prostate cancer. There are no published experiments proving the cancer specific efficacy of surgery or radiotherapy against an adequate, autochthonous[454] prostate cancer animal model. Autochthonous means that the cancer arose from the animal's own tissues; it is not a transplant from some other animal or species. This distinction is important because effects alleged to be the result of therapy can easily be the result of immune rejection of foreign tissues if the tumor is not autocthonous.

In the history of the world, there is only one series of experiments regarding the efficacy of surgery for prostate cancer in whole animals.[455] They showed that surgery alone, without chemotherapy, 'cures' fifty percent of the rats when the volume of the implant is below eight tenths of a cubic centimeter. But these experiments were not even close to the situation in man. This is 200 times the usual volume, 004 cc's (2 mm in diameter), at which metastases from solid tumors usually begin. In this model, the implanted cancer (not autocthonous) was clearly having a harder time metastasizing than cancers usually do. It suggests that only in a condition of antigen (chemical groups on the cell surface to which the animal is allergic) excess can this model thrive. Most human cancers including prostate cancer inspire no immune response. Even without that criticism, the model rebuts the putative efficacy of radical prostatectomy in man because, at half of the 2.5 cubic centimeters found in the radical prostatectomy specimens of men without elevated PSAs, it still allows two years of metastases to occur prior to radical prostatectomy. See the chapter on bone marrow metastases.

There are other problems with this model: (1) such a volume, proportioned to man's weight, would be two hundred cubic centimeters and would occur after 12 years of metastases and four years before death; (2) the Dunning tumor cells have a two and a half day doubling time in a rat's life time of two years; when calculated to be proportionate to a human life time of 75 years, that represents a seventy-eight day doubling time, an average figure for human cancer like breast, but less than a quarter of the four hundred and seventy-five day figure determined by the Johns Hopkins group for human prostate cancer; (3) worst of all, the Dunning tumor is not prostatic in origin; it metastasizes to lung instead of bone marrow. Prostate cancer does not thrive in lung, Max Lerner's peculiar experience and one recently published case notwithstanding.

The Nobelist, Andrew Schally, described in Chapter 11, has spent his life since the prize on experimental prostate cancer models. He now only uses actual human prostate cancers, e.g. DU145 androgen independent, implanted in nude mice. These mice are immune deficient. This is better but it is still a graft from one species to another. Prof.

Schally has sextupled this tumor's doubling time from 32.1 days to 184 days with an elegant antihormone drug of his invention. Tumor weight was lowered sixty-eight percent.[456] This is biology direct, and supports the thesis of this book that the proper therapy of prostate cancer is systemic from the get-go.

There is actually no lack of bench research on prostate cancer in the universities. A Medline search for "prostate cancer, animal models" yields nine pages of references. They are, alas, not helpful for the clinician. The references are all about prostate cancer cells growing in a dish, tissue culture. One can understand why there are no prostatectomy studies in the mouse. However, cancer of the prostate has been identified in the dog. Surely it would be possible to do a radical prostatectomy or radiation in a dog! There are no references. An ocean of tissue culture studies has done nothing to interrupt the tide of radical surgery and radiotherapy in the whole man preparation. Tissue culture is too far from medical care to affect practice.

An additional reason that 'bench' evidence, hard science, has lost its punch in medical schools is the decline of the autopsies performed by the Departments of Pathology in the United States. Until after World War II, a year of pathology could take the place of a year with the animals at the bench in the biography of a future professor of medicine. Clinicians headed for academic medicine did autopsies. Now, the rates are below 5%. The reasons are: no direct reimbursement to the hospital for the activity, fear of litigation if a discrepancy is found between the autopsy and the clinical diagnosis, and increased diagnostic accuracy with endoscopes and computerized tomography.[457] Diagnostic error has, in fact, been cut in half in the past 20 years. But what has been lost has been a constant reminder in formal morbidity and mortality conferences of the frequency of incidental cancers of all kinds including occult, incidental prostate and thyroid cancers, not to mention the reality of occasional deaths as a consequence of surgery, *e.g.* Professor Gilbert in California.

In addition to Medicare and the bootless trend to research in a dish instead of whole animals, the post 1960s trend toward more electives in the medical school curriculum facilitated the epidemic.[458] In the 1960s, 80% of medical schools required a rotation through urology. By 1990, only 20% did. Medical students were encouraged by the French deconstructionists and Ivan Illych to think that the academic hierarchy knew little of use and that they, the students, could calculate priorities about medicine and surgery well even before studying the topic. The students have tended to choose the romantic electives shown on television like emergency room work, neurosurgery, or cardiac surgery over urology. I do not believe a rectal exam for prostate cancer has ever been depicted on network television. It is hard to find advertisers for that.

The sum of the vectors above has been away from the bench as described in Claude Bernard's Introduction to Experimental Medicine and toward an ever foggier, normative, uniform, clinical experience resembling a pre-Flexner, University of London model. Contemporary clinical experience is not directed by the results of animal science in the lab. It is governed clinical consensus statements requested by the third party payers like Medicare, private insurers and the malpractice carriers. These statements are eagerly provided by specialty societies and are self-serving. These cookbooks are, in turn, based incestuously but fashionably on clinical experience, not animal experimentation. The consensus statements are supposed to say what you should do but in fact only record what M.D.s are doing. Current medical students and resident trainees are forced by vast unpaid student loans to do what everybody ahead of them is doing to earn a living. Students, at least in the case of many solid cancers, often would do just as well to go to the Kalahari Desert and join a circle around a campfire with the click people to find out the consensus.

The problem of consensus statements is illustrated by 1995 American Urological Association (A.U.A.) policy statement on the management of apparently localized prostate cancer previously addressed in Chapter 13. The first half was solidly evidence based but the second half was not; it was consensus based. This dichotomy should have been made clear but was not. Consensus is level 5, the lowest, on the "quality of evidence" hierarchy.[459] What is called level 1 evidence; multiple, prospective, controlled, randomized clinical trials with similar findings, is hugely expensive. Nobody has yet spent the necessary money in the case of radical surgery or radiation for a proper study of prostate cancer. The A.U.A. panel avoided condemnation of the epidemic because of this lack of evidence. It generated the fog of consensus which hid the troops advancing toward profit. The 2007 revision has not changed that.

Consensus based medical care is not in the tradition of medicine and surgery in which I was raised. My grandfather, John Rogers, graduated from Columbia P&S in 1892, an exciting time when the curriculum, even before Flexner's report, began to be based, not on consensus, but rather on Claude Bernard's experimental medicine in animals. For years, Dr. Rogers supported at his own expense a lab technician at New York Cornell Medical Center who assisted him in his Bernardian investigations while he earned a living caring for the worried well of Park Avenue. My mother told me that his independent streak caused plenty of professional jealousy. He died in 1939, two months before I was born. Even so, when I followed him to Columbia's College of Physicians and Surgeons (P&S) sixty-nine years later, I thought that every practicing clinician in the trenches, not just salaried, full-time employees of medical schools, should have a hard science bench project on going.

I have to admit that the over zealous application of the Columbia P&S/Flexner tradition can bear strange fruit. When, as surgical resident, I acquired bacteria in my blood from a laboratory rat, a Columbia P&S graduate internist handling my hospital admission steadfastly refused to give me an antibiotic until the laboratory had identified the organism. It turned out to be an unusual organism usually found in the blood of Bowery bums bitten by rats but exquisitely sensitive to penicillin. Another P&S graduate who was training to be a pathologist in that very laboratory was incensed that I had not been given an antibiotic as soon as the cultures had been drawn. He was worried about my developing bacterial growth in the sac around my brain or on my heart valves while we waited for the creatures to grow out in culture. With thirty years of experience as an M.D., I now side with the second P&S graduate, the pathology trainee. The internist had confused Bernardian, pre-clinical, bench science with its application, bedside medicine. He should have, after taking all manner of cultures, filled me on that first day with an antibiotic or two. The Flexner/Columbia P&S tradition of scientific medicine can be overdone.

Or underdone. A key fact about 'Flexner' medical schools between 1920 and 1965 is that Departments of Internal Medicine saw themselves as the guardians of scientific (now called evidence-based) medicine. They were arbiters of whether or not a surgeon should even be consulted. Surgeons (urology evolved out of general surgery) made big money, internists much less. Internists feuded bitterly with them because of envy of their income. Internists could (and did) choke off the livelihood of surgeons they thought were doing unnecessary procedures. I remember seeing this during my straight medical internship of 1965-66.

But this Appalachian feud was beginning to moderate at the same time and not for a good reason. Internal medicine residents were beginning to do the cardiac catheterization procedures pioneered by two salaried, full-timers on the City of New York's payroll, Andre Cournand and Dickinson Richards of Columbia's Bellevue division. More recently, cardiologists have been putting stents in the coronaries. Every once in a while they need to be rescued by an immediate 'open' procedure by a cardiac surgeon. Open feuds between the two specialties would be bad for business. Internists on renal fellowships in those days probed blindly for the kidney, identified it by feel, and then took a core to identify the various kinds of cellular disease. Sometimes the kidney bled and they needed to call a urologist. If the urologist consulted challenged the necessity of the biopsy, he would receive no more consults from the nephrologists. By the late 1960s, internists trained in gastroenterology sent long fiberoptic tubes down the esophagus and up the colon. They took biopsies which sometimes perforated the colon and needed an open general surgical procedure immediately. They too could not afford to be at war with general surgery nor general surgery with them. They had come to rely on procedures, not evaluation and management, for their income which sky-rocketed. All the insurance plans including Medicare and Medicaid pay more for procedures. Internists have been massively engaged in surgery since the 1970s. Now it is, "You scratch my back and I'll scratch yours."

Immense sums of money from the federal and state governments flowed into internal medicine departments in university medical schools. I rented part of my office space to a gastroenterologist who had just graduated from his training program at Beth Israel in Manhattan in the late 1970s. After a month or two, he moved out saying he could make more profit doing two colonoscopies in the hospital than he could working a whole day in the office. Subspecialty internists began to fly to small towns on the high plains like locusts to do procedures. When I was recruited as a urologist to Lander, Wyoming, in the late 1980s, I learned of a gastroenterologist who flew up bi-weekly from New Orleans to do colonoscopies. The money was worth it.

Internal medicine has never developed the quasi-military discipline to govern these procedures that characterizes university hospital surgical departments in regard to formal operations in operating rooms. Consider general surgery's traditional death and complications conference. I remember, as a resident, hearing a senior attending state his apprehension at an upcoming conference. The best of them, like a good military officer, did not conceal but rather owned up to their errors. They had an honesty which earned the respect of the trainees because the trainee would not be routed out of bed in the middle of the night for the same complication twice. Surgery is a deeply cooperative business like warfare. Surgery, in fact, arose from warfare *e.g.* Stephen Maturin, M.D. of the Patrick O'Brien's series of novels about the Napoleonic wars. By contrast, internal medicine arose from universities, not the battlefield. It was when I graduated in 1965 more cerebral, freer of procedures, and their contaminating large sums of money.

Not now. Internists now are doing procedures but with a difference from their surgical counterparts. They do not use formally designated operating rooms. Gastroenterologists work in something called G.I. lab with a looser set of rules. This is how they escape the military discipline sketched above. They also give their own sedation and so escape the critical eye of anesthesiologists. They have no tradition of a death and complications conference. Death is so routine and so often the result of the patient's disease on internal medicine that one more following a procedure excites little interest.

There is one more faction in the medical polity that used to have a policeman's function, radiology. It was they who spotted the clamp left in the belly. I remember one at my internship hospital who stopped an operation that would have cut off the leg of a twenty year old. There was said to be a cancer at the insertion of his hamstring muscle on his pelvis. The night before the operation was to occur, one of the radiologists looked at the films and read them as compatible with repair of a disruption of the insertion of the hamstring on the pelvis. The young man, in retrospect, gave a history of a sudden pain when practicing for the hop, step, and jump competition. The operation was cancelled. The radiologist had saved a leg but the surgeon and the hospital had lost money.

Being right on a diagnosis that cancels an operation is not the hot thing in radiology anymore. It pays little and makes enemies. What is hot is doing surgery without the hard work of five years of residency in a department of surgery. With the help of computerized tomography, ultrasound, and fluoroscopy, radiologists are doing all kinds of procedures previously done by surgeons and being well paid for it. This is called interventional radiology. They start at $350,000 per year. Some of them are doing parts of my specialty without the required year of general surgery and a four year residency with six months to a year in the lab that the urologic specialty board requires. The public has lost radiology as a referee in a vast economic *sauve qui peut*, a rout.

The reader needs to understand that the organized medical staff of a university hospital is a separate organization from the university medical school faculty. The by-laws of the medical staff place a high value on collegiality. Indeed, a M.D. can be kicked off the medical staff of a hospital simply for not being sufficiently collegiate, never mind whether he is right scientifically. He is called disruptive and is subject to discipline of his license by the state medical board. Under this circumstance, there is no reward for blowing a whistle on any of the many doubtful procedures that earn money for the university hospital and the faculty practice plan, much less radical surgery and radiotherapy for prostate cancer. Just as the savings and loan debacle occurred because of a law passed by Congress and signed by the President (cash for trash), so also does the epidemic of prostate cancer care continue to be driven by immense, legal, sums of money in a free market economy. Mammon reins in university hospital administration as it must if they are to survive inflation.

Not to overstate the case, Plato's shadow of the ideal scientific doctor is still being projected on the walls of Columbia's P&S, the University of Chicago,[460] Vanderbilt, Stanford, the University of Iowa, and several others of the older, more conservative, medical schools. They continue to produce the self-reliant, crusty, ornery, incorruptible, laboratory grounded specialist I imagine my grandfather to have been. However, at some of the expansion medical schools founded in the 1970s[461] and at the satellite, residency training programs not directly attached to their parent universities, the Flexner vision is not cherished. It is thought to be elitist. In my opinion, the United States standard of care, a not-so-fictional construct of malpractice lawyers and third party payers, is not set by the graduates and trainees of the medical schools on Flexner's A list. It is set by the graduates of the expansion schools and training programs founded to take care of the immense demand for free medical care stimulated by Medicare/Medicaid. They are far more numerous than 'Flexner' graduates. Even the 'Flexner' graduates are not a homogeneous crew. Many have not bought into his vision. At one point, Abraham Flexner urged the Rockefellers' General Education Board to sue my alma mater, Columbia's P&S, for backsliding on full-time, *i.e.* allowing fees from private practice to accrue to professors supposedly living on bonds bought with Rockefeller money.

In my opinion, the widespread, Medicare inspired, undeclared bankruptcies of the medical school associated hospitals characteristic of the period 1983 to the present, plus the change in the composition of the M.D. workforce, plus the re-orientation of internal medicine and radiology toward procedures, plus the loss of the department of pathology as a disciplinarian through autopsies has caused the widespread erosion of Flexner's ideals both in the university and community hospitals. Additional vectors were/are (1) the shortage of M.D.s trained at the bench work (2) the ravenous, Johnsonian inflation which destroyed the valued of endowed professorships based on the income from bonds. These vectors permitted our two atavistic but remunerative procedures, radical prostatectomy and radiation for alleged 'cure,' to slip under the radar. There was only a muted, brief outcry from the Flexner supported University of Chicago and the full-time Memorial Sloan-Kettering derived from General Motors money in New York. The Flexner schools have been mostly silent or active promoters of radical surgery and radiation for alleged 'cure.'

The high road followed by my grandfather, John Rogers, M.D., at Cornell Medical School 1895 to 1938 has been flooded. One hears an occasional shout above the churning commercial waters. For example, H. Ballentine Carter at Johns Hopkins, quoted my paper on the mean time to death for cancers of the sort discovered by PSA in the November, 2003, issue of the United States journal, Urology.[462] He seemed to be signaling that he is a foe of the epidemic of care. But in general, the stern visaged chairmen of medicine and surgery salaried via the interest from bonds have been unhorsed. Emerson's 'things' have got back into the university medical school 'saddle.' The United States medical schools have regressed to their nineteenth century, proprietary, business mode.[463] That is why they did not stop, have not stopped, an epidemic of prostate cancer case finding, surgery, and radiation unsupported by science.

We need a new Flexner report. Kenneth Ludmerer's history of American medical education since the Flexner report is a start. Maybe some future president will nudge the university hospitals toward science-based medical care.

CHAPTER 17

Medicine as a business.

"...Many men with clinically insignificant microfoci of disease are currently being diagnosed, and the CaPSURE data confirm that more than 90% of these men are being treated radically."—Laurence Klotz, American Urological Association News, Nov. 2007

W hy is this? How can Laurence Klotz be right in a country devoted to science? The answer is that the United States is devoted to business more.

My lifetime covers the defeat of fascism and communism. The first was obliterated by fire and sword, the second by bankruptcy. The United States has demonstrated, according to C.E. Lindblom, a third way in which society may be governed, that is by the sum total of its commercial entities, its businesses. He explored the idea of business as a form of government in a 1977 book called *Politics And Markets: The World's Political Economic Systems.* My reading of it started the political science education I had neglected in college.

At that time, I had just entered the private practice of medicine in New York City. My main hospital was a Catholic hospital on the west side of Manhattan, St. Clare's. New York City had just flirted with economic disaster which was averted by the issuance of what were called Big Mac Bonds. The bonds had been bought by the retirement plans for hospital workers offered by the Health and Hospital Corporation, the partially privatized municipal hospital system. In the post 1965 Medicaid/Medicare era, they were supposed to be self-supporting via fee-for-service but the umbilical cord had never really been cut. The New York City and State taxpayers continued to subsidize a massive skein of socialized medicine.

In those days in New York State, hospitals had to petition the state to (1) raise the daily rate of hospital inpatients or (2) to add a service or a piece of capital equipment. This was called a Certificate of Need and it was state socialism. As secretary to the county medical society, I was able to sit in on meetings with New York State officials.

From this vantage point, I saw that, when hospitals in the municipal system asked for a raise in their daily room rate or a new piece of equipment, they got it. By contrast, when private sector hospitals such as mine asked, they did not.

The power of the State was impressive. My hospital or any other, no matter how well established or well endowed, could be squashed like a bug by the State of New York. For example, when New York Hospital furnished and endowed a new burn unit, they were denied a Certificate of Need. The state regulators said burn patients should go to a municipal hospital, Bellevue, which had a burn unit. This way money from private sector insurance policies was directed into municipal coffers to shore up the municipal pension plans. The Health and Hospitals Corporation had bought Big Mac bonds as part of the city's plan to emerge from undeclared bankruptcy and they needed the money.

Hospitals are critical for me as a surgeon. But hospital administration in New York City was a murky mix of the three elements explored by Lindblom, *i.e.* free market, socialism, and government by persuasion. He called such a mixture "market socialism" and pointed to Yugoslavia and Hungary as evolving models worth emulating. He was fond of this middle ground between free market and government, because he had determined that the modern corporation did not fit into democratic theory. The corporations in the United States were too politically powerful, he thought, to be controlled by the regulatory agencies in place. In 2008, we had learned that our major corporation may not be that strong, that they may go bankrupt in a heartbeat.

His book looks woefully out of date now. Yugoslavia is in ethnic shards. Central Europe has gone the free market route only to be ambushed by a worldwide credit crisis. Adam Smith's invisible hand of capitalism appears to be non-existent when major brokerage houses self-destruct. But what would Lindblom's angle of vision made of the epidemic of prostate cancer care? Did our government, which footed the bill for perhaps 80% of the epidemic, have sufficient regulatory power to bring it to a halt? Where do we place medical care in the United States on Linblom's spectrum of regulation by government versus regulation by market forces? What should be done, if anything, about the prostate cancer epidemic as a public health matter?

I received more education about the business/government intersection when I worked part-time for Blue Cross Blue Shield of New York during those same private practice days, 1980-1983. Our job was to develop policy about what should be paid for, how much to pay, and what should not be paid for by Blue Cross Blue Shield and Medicare. I remember when the decision to pay for penile prostheses arrived on my desk from Washington. I was happy with the coverage decision as a urologist but, as a citizen, I was appalled. I wrote to the Washington D.C. Medicare headquarters protesting that a guarantee of permanent erections for the Medicare population would put an unlimited raid on the taxpayer's wallet. I got back a memo stating that cost was not an issue under the Medicare statute; medical necessity was the only issue. I was writing policy for a federal program without spending brakes.

My alarm was strengthened when I learned at committee meetings that Blue Cross Blue Shield N.Y., as a Medicare carrier, won its contract with the federal government on its costs per claim. The total cost of the program was not and is not a factor in winning a contract with the Medicare administration in Washington. This non-profit corporation was merely a conduit for cash flow. It would retain or lose its contract with the Feds according to the friction generated by the flow, not the aggregate volume of the flow. This was true of the various Medicare carriers throughout the country. All were private corporations with government contracts similar to the model for the production of tanks in World War II by General Motors. The Russians in World War II had state run tank factories that were not nearly as good as our private sector outsourcing model.

Thus, Medicare in the 1980s did not represent the triumph of socialism. To pass the Medicare law through the Congress in 1965 during the middle of the Cold War, the bill's managers made it resemble free-market capitalism, not Russian communism. Thomas Friedman, a columnist for the New York Times, refers to free market capitalism as a locomotive with nobody in the engineer's cab. And so it has proved to be in the case of prostate cancer as well as the international credit debacle of 2008.

I learned, as I worked at Blue Cross Blue Shield of N.Y. (B.C.B.S.N.Y.), that the commonest rationale for paying for a procedure by a Medicare carrier was the fact that another Blue Cross Blue Shield plan or Medicare carrier had decided to pay for it. The library of this non-profit corporation did not carry any peer reviewed medical journals. It carried only insurance industry trade journals and books. A payment policy, called coverage, grew by echoes between the various Blue Cross Blue Shield plans around the country not by reference to human biology. To this day coverage decisions are capricious. I successfully changed a coverage decision when practicing in Wyoming but it took a lot of time for which I was not paid.

Eventually, in the case of radiation and surgery for prostate cancer, the Medicare administration did react to the aggregate system wide cost through its research wing in Kansas City. This occurred in 1993, one year after the frequency of the surgical operations peaked and five years after the American Urological Association had formed its committee on the scientific basis of the epidemic. From 1993 to 1997, because of pressure from peer review organizations, local M.D.s working as Medicare policemen, the upward slope of radical prostatectomies performed per 100,000 beneficiaries turned negative, and flattened in the over age 75 group.[464] See Figure 1.

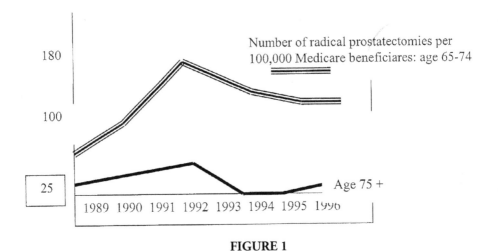

FIGURE 1

Utilization of radical prostatectomy 1986-1996. Medicare announced an investigation of the sudden increase in surgery from 1987 to 1992. Their announcement caused an immediate decrease after 1992. It has continued to decrease after 2011 because two randomized, prospective, controlled studies have showed no significant life extension compared to no treatment.

Part of the explanation for the improvement in the death rate since 1992 is the abrupt decline in the over age 75 group targeted by the Kansas City bureaucrats. It is these surgical elderly that were dying in large numbers of postoperative clots in their coronaries and lungs. These deaths were ascribed to prostate cancer improperly instead of the complications of major surgery.

This decline is an example of Lindblom's government regulation by persuasion. In this case, government carried a pretty big stick in the form of its ability to kick an M.D. out of the Medicare program and put his name in the local paper as having been dropped. This would destroy the livelihood of almost all physicians. Sheik and Bullock, the authors who implemented this campaign against the radical prostatectomy, did not believe that their federal government effort had had any effect at all when I corresponded with them. I believe they were wrong: the announcement of their intent to scrutinize the epidemic had a powerful effect. So did a peer reviewed critique of the operation which was published in 1993 in the Journal of the American Medical Association.[465] Private practitioners needed only the announcement of the government's intention to study a topic to change their ways. Unfortunately, by 1995-96 the Kansas City Feds effect had begun to weaken and radical prostatectomy rates began to rise again.

Other forces emanating from the existing social capital of the country must have been at work beside the Feds to cause the downturn and plateau at a lower level. Fukuyama says that humans predictably re-assert order when faced with prolonged disorder. Among the privately insured citizens of Olmstead county, MN, home of the Mayo Clinic, the dramatic increase in the rate of radical prostatectomies faltered as early as 1990 in the 70-79 age group, and a year later in the 60-69 age group. This may have been an effect of the establishment in1987 of the American Urological Association Panel to study the problem of why the sudden rise in radical prostatic surgery and radiation in the absence of new published evidence of life extension.

In 2009, the entire country became more homogeneous in its use of radical prostatic surgery. The Northeast and Mid-Atlantic states have capitulated to the epidemic and are doing more radical surgery. This could be the result of pressure from the urology residency review committee. This committee can put a urology residency in jeopardy if it does not see enough radical prostatectomies. The Mountain and Pacific states are performing fewer radicals. But there is no reason to relax our vigilance because, when brachytherapy, radioactive seeding, was added to radical surgery, the total number of treatments with intent to cure had almost returned to the 1992 peak in 1997.[466] In some areas of the country, brachytherapy far exceeds radical surgery. Androgen deprivation therapy, with which I agree, rose dramatically in response to unrealistically high reimbursement by Medicare and then declined when the reimbursement was equated to cost plus 10%. I and others ascribe much of the current decline in the death rate from prostate cancer to the increase in early androgen deprivation therapy.

In the case of pills, injections, and implanted artificial devices, the United States Food and Drug Administration (F.D.A.) demands evidence before it approves the label. For example in 2003 there was a lengthy hearing on whether or not to allow breast implants containing silicon gel back on the market. The F.D.A. measures effectiveness versus risk. In the case of breast implant, one witness testified that without any measurable benefit there could be no safety. Under this standard approval, both radical prostatectomy and radiation would not pass the F.D.A. But the F.D.A. is not authorized to disapprove operations and radiation sources. While I think vast sums are being wasted, I am not willing to cede the government more power to judge the admissibility of surgical operations. They will never, as Lindblom copiously illustrated among the communists, get it right. This is why Russian communism went bankrupt. No government agency is smart enough to make the right decision at this level of detail. A very imperfect market will decide. It is deciding it but it is doing it too slowly.

Government, via Medicare, has begun to regulate the frequency of surgical operations by controlling the level of reimbursement. It appears to me as a private practitioner that in recent years the financial reward for radical prostatectomy has become so low, $1300, that the incentive for radical surgery at the community level, with its attendant calls in the night, is lost. This may be the reason urologists are steering the citizens toward seeds instead. But note well that it is not only the surgical fee that draws urologists to the operation. Equity ownership of the means of production, the O.R. suite, is increasingly common. In early 2004, 28% of urologists had financial interest in an ambulatory surgical center.[467]

Even androgen deprivation is big business. The $2,000 that TAP pharmaceuticals used to receive every three months for medical androgen deprivation per patient has caused some urologists to be convicted of a felony. These urologists were selling at full price to Medicare the medicine they were given for free as samples. The manufacturer of the competing medicine, Zoladex, "pleaded guilty to violating a federal drug marketing law and will pay $35,000,000 to settle allegations of illegal pricing and marketing of the prostate cancer drug Zoladex...In addition to giving Zoladex to physicians who charged patients and insurance programs for the samples, the FDA said, the company inflated the price of Zoladex reported to Medicare as the basis for reimbursement."[468]

Identifying prostate cancer metastases is big business. A medical article in the New England Journal of Medicine (NEJM) regarding the identification of metastases prior to localized therapy with intent to cure sparked a sudden jump in the share price of Advanced Magnetics a few days before the appearance of the print addition would make the information public knowledge. It turns out that about 350 members of the media and all the subscribers, which included me, received the article a few days before the print edition appeared. James R. Ferguson, a partner in the Chicago law firm of Mayer Brown, *et al*, found no restriction on NEJM subscribers trading on the information before the print edition.[469] Many traded. I did not. The stock went up 39%, and volume increased eight times its daily average before the print edition appeared. Nothing illegal here. Just business as usual.

Capital equipment for prostate cancer is also big business. A chairman of urology in a major university long active in prostate cancer research got caught up in the commercial frenzy of the 1990s and lost his title, his job, and, briefly his medical license, over double dipping on travel claims. But that was only the tip of the iceberg; he had extolled on the scientific podium and in print the excellence of ultrasound equipment manufactured by a corporation in which he served as a member of the board of directors without revealing his conflict of interest. This was like Henry Blogett of Merrill Lynch pumping up dot.com stocks that were also investment banking clients. The urology chairman is now former and is currently not listed as a member of the American Urological Association nor is he any longer the editor of one of the two major U.S. journals of urology.

Since just about everybody in American medicine was involved in the business of prostatic surgery and radiation, I do not fault the individual urologist/radiation oncologist in his private office much as I cannot find fault with those who did not join the French resistance in World War II. It is a hard life to contest the culture. Thirty percent of us urologists in the West still work solo down from 46% when I first came to the Far West. We exist in a whirlpool of money that we did not invent. Urologists/radiation oncologists need to pay their student loans, their mortgage rent, their malpractice insurance, their children's college tuition, and to fund their retirement. If somebody is referred to a urologist by a non-specialist because of an elevated prostatic specific antigen laboratory report, the die is cast. Most urologists will do what he is expected to do by Mr. Market. As a solo private practitioner and, therefore, a small businessman once again, I do not see any of my suppliers, my insurers, my power generators, or my landlords lowering their prices because they are making too much money. I do not see medical school or hospital business expenses going down. I do not see my son's private college lowering their tuition. I see administrators everywhere in Gucchi shoes.

Even worse, insurance companies in recent years have engaged in gangster-like activities to deprive their insured customers of coverage for their doctor's bills. They take the premiums and do not pay the M.D. timely or at all has been the practice. 950,000 active and retired physicians sued Aetna under the RICCO statute designed for organized crime in a class action. On December 3rd, 2003, a U.S. district judge in Miami approved an Aetna settlement offer[470] of 100 million dollars to reimburse doctors for denied claims, 50 million dollars in legal fees, and 300 million dollars to overhaul its claims processing systems and improve communication with physicians. When I was in private practice in the early 1980s, the head of the local Blue Cross Blue Shield boasted to a newspaper reporter that he delayed sending out reimbursement checks to the M.D.s for months in order to earn more interest in the bank. This was my world. The trend is for more consolidation in the insurance industry to get rid of what John D. Rockefeller called "ruinous competition." United Health, a monopoly in some regions, one of them southwest Wyoming where I worked for four years, is the darling of Wall Street even though its recently departed founder and CEO backdated his stock options.

Reasonable therapies are kept from the U.S. public because of over-regulation by the Federal Drug Administration. This happened to the first proven immune therapy for prostate cancer, Provenge. The drug which was really the patient's own white cells instructed to chase/kill cells containing prostatic acid phosphatase was denied approval at first. This denial immensely increased the cost of development. Provenge was finally approved in April, 2010. But the manufacturing corporation, Dendreon, filed for bankruptcy in November, 2014. The following year, 2015, all Dendreon assets were approved for purchase by Valeant Pharmaceuticals. But this was a shaky arrangement too because Valeant immediately raised the price over $100,000 for a series of three treatments.

I think that licensed M.D.s should be able to exercise their four years of graduate education and four more of on the job training. Let them be their own FDA. This is not a dangerous poison. The Feds just don't want to pay for it under Medicare.

Private practice urologists are corks in a free-market sea. A principled stand against a therapy which yields good money can sink them as competitive business entities. Full-timers in academia are not much better off. Their salaries are 80% funded by revenue from private practice. The part of their income derived from state tax money in the state sponsored schools such as U.C.S.F., where I had an academic appointment, has not been reliable. California escaped bankruptcy via a bond issue. In 2008, it had to write to the U.S. treasury for a bridge loan. During my entire thirty-eight years as an M.D., the issue of who-will-pay-the-M.D.-how-much has been up for grabs. Often nobody pays. I was stiffed in Wyoming by a recently released prisoner with $6.00 to his name. I put out labor and expendables but nothing came back. We bob in a sea of unfunded mandates. We must take care of patients who show up unstable in the emergency room. They pay nothing. If they are referred to me while I am under contract to the hospital, I must take care of them. This is called the EMTALA rule. It is the slavery outlawed by Lincoln. It embodies the belief among many that somehow the M.D. need not be paid anything. During the period of the early epidemic, 1986 to 2002, when I had a salary from the federal government that allowed me to resist Adam Smith's invisible hand, the for-profit sector was pre-occupied with economic survival. Science has been a luxury fee-for-service docs could ill afford.

CHAPTER 18

The Confidence Game weakens after the US Preventive Task Force (USPTF) statement in 2012.

As stated in the preface, the prostate cancer paradigm inverted in 2012 when the USPTF declared that PSA based screening did more harm than good. Frendl, D. et al reported insurance claims data in the July 2016 AUA News which showed a steady state of percent eligible men screened from 2000 to 2010 in Massachusetts. But the percent drops -26% in the ages 55-69, 2010-2013, after the USPTF announcement. Jemal, A. of the American Cancer Society reported a lesser, 7%, decline in screening PSAs from 2010-2013 in ages 50-74 in SEER registries from all over the United States, quite different from Massachusetts as a famously liberal, democratic state, responsive to science.

There has been wide variation between the various states' responses to the USPSTF as reported by Firas Abdollah of Michigan et al at the annual spring meeting of the AUA in 2016. While Alabama and Alaska had the highest drop, 7.5%, in PSA screening, Utah had virtually no change in screening practice. Vermont was similar to Alaska and Alabama. So, the response of United States primary care to the USPTF declaration was patchy. Overall, less screening occurred in 2013 compared to 2012.

USPSTF relied on two studies of screening to make their decision. The United States study, PLCO, was itself studied and turned out to be a comparison of regularly timed PSA screening versus ad hoc irregular PSA screening. PSA enthusiasts cried 'foul' but anti-screeners thought that the data showed no difference and was not supportive of screening. Gerald L. Andriole, M.D., Robert K. Royce, distinguished professor and Chief of Urologic Surgery, Washington University School of Medicine, was one of the authors of the US PLCO report. He showed slides to the January 2016 International Prostate Cancer Update (IPCU) in Vail, Colorado, that supported the USPTF decision to give screening with PSA a 'D.' An early slide said, "Mass population screening has a small effect on CaP mortality (3% to 2.1%)" and I would add, "within the 10 year follow up period." He also said of PLCO, "no benefit for entire group." Later in the talk he said that, "in the PIVOT trial of screen-detected cancers…no overall benefit" with the caution that using an action value of PSA>10 does produce benefit, a key observation.

Prof. Andriole also reported the apparent benefit of the European study of screening, ERSPC, as "-20-30% RR (relative risk reduction of death) in a subgroup." Richard J. Ablin, PhD, discoverer of the PSA molecule, and author (with Ronald Piana) of *The Great Prostate Hoax*, published an op-ed piece in the New York Times for November 11, 2014 stating several methodological flaws in ERSPC: (1) the Swedish Goteberg study's authors would not allow outside investigators to study their data; (2) Ian E.Haines and George L. Gabor Miklos pointed out that "a large amount of the data in ERSPC came from a separately reported Finnish study that showed no significant lifesaving benefits of PSA Screening"; (3) excessive hormonal monotherapy; (4) the non-screened Swedish men were not informed they were in a clinical trial; and (5) several senior authors had potential conflicts of interest. The pro-screening faction has clung to the European study as a 'life raft' for their increased income but it was finally discredited, in my opinion, at the annual meeting of the AUA in San Diego, May 6, 2016. There, Monique J. Roobol of the Netherlands et al showed that the apparent improvement of the relative risk of death during the study period by PSA screening in Europe was "caused by detecting cancer at an earlier stage and grade," i.e. lead time bias. In 2018, the USPTF succumbed to pressure from the pro-screening faction and changed its 'D' to 'C' to screening from 55 to 69. But, a 'C' still means that the Medicare private sector carriers need not pay for PSA for screening. A 'C' is faint praise. So far, they all have continued to pay.

The true demise of stand alone PSA screening occurred later on October 26th at 11:20 a.m., 2016, at the annual meeting of the Western Section of the AUA in Kauai, Hawaii where Peter Carroll, M.D., professor, and chairman at UCSF held the affirmative that, "Early detection of prostate cancer with serum PSA needs to be refined" while William Catalona, M.D., of Northwestern, Chicago, was supposed to hold the negative. It was Prof. Catalona who had argued with the FDA on August 25, 1994 for the indication of stand alone PSA for cancer screening years after it had been approved for monitoring known cancers. His testimony at that time was self-contradicting but sufficiently emotional to sway some members. But faced with Prof. Carrol's eloquent oral critique of screening with stand-alone PSA in October 2016, he capitulated in front of the Western Section and suggested that as a standard, we should do more PSA densities, i.e. divide the PSA by the prostate volume. Thirty years before, Mitchell Benson, M.D., had shown that if the density is <.15, the elevation may reliably be ascribed to BPH; and the cancer scare is off. I did densities starting in 1987 to get rid of the false positives caused by the action value of 4 ug/dl. Prof. Catalona's podium statement about the utility of PSA density did not appear on his slides for a prostate cancer course given earlier in the week. In his 1994 testimony to the FDA quoted in Prof. Ablin's *The Great Prostate Hoax* (pg. 83) he says, "PSA is a more powerful predictor of prostate cancer than rectal examination." Notice that the 'PSA' he touts is unmodified; he did not say to use the PSA number to compute density.

With the decline of PSA screening, ablative therapies have gone into a sharp decline. Katherine Rotker et al of Providence RI reported at the AUA 2016 annual meeting a 35% decline in radical prostatectomies after the 2012 USPTF pronouncement. Kathleen McGinley of Binghamton N.Y., Martha K. Terris, Chairman and Professor of Urology at Augusta, Georgia, et al, (five of the others work as I do in the far west of the U.S.) reported at the same meeting that the percent receiving radical prostatectomy of their series of low risk disease went from 42% in the 1994-1999 period to 13% in the 2014-2015 period. This probably represents a large drop in absolute numbers of operations for the whole and therefore money to the faculty practice plan because screening with PSA does its best job when it discovers clinically insignificant disease, i.e. Gleason 6 and below. As is typical of the western appetite for action, western urologists reported a 20% increase in radical prostatectomies in intermediate risk men and a 9% increase in high risk men. But, I suspect that absolute numbers of radical prostatectomies are significantly down for the whole group. This would cause a considerable loss of top line receipts just as Theragenics, a radioactive seed company, reported its first loss in the first quarter of 2013 after the USPSTF notice of May, 2012, and was forced to sell itself to a larger corporation. See Chapter 9.

But sharp declines in radical prostatectomies did not occur uniformly over the USA. Where I live and practiced, the southern San Joaquin Valley of California, showed only a 3% decline in radical prostatectomies, 2012-13, despite a 30% decline in making the diagnosis, 2009-2013. A large private urology practice in Dallas, TX, reported in 2016 at the AUA annual meeting no declines either in the diagnosis (PSAs drawn/biopsies) or radical prostatectomy rates.

Declines similar to those in radical prostatectomy/brachytherapy have occurred in external beam radiation business. M. Cooperburg and P. Carroll, both M.D. and M.P.H., reported in the July, 2015, JAMA, a 10% drop in % low risk patients receiving radiation from the 2005-2009 cohort to the 2010-2013 post USPSTF cohort. -3-7% changes occurred in the middle and high risk classifications. While these are not decreases like radical prostatectomy (-16% overall in U.S.A. according to Halpern et al. in JAMA Surg. 2017) they may be fatal for the high capitalization, debt/interest rate businesses like the Winthrop Cyberknife, an affiliate of the NYU Langone Hospital in Manhattan. A full page ad for this cyberknife has appeared in every Sunday N.Y. Times magazine section during 2016-17. They tout similar rates of success to radical surgery but the latter, of course, is no better than no treatment controls.

These negative rates for radical prostatectomy and external beam were also caused by the increased enthusiasm for prostate cancer surveillance started in 2002 by Prof. of Urology, Lawrence Klotz, M.D., of Canada. It was his 'surveillance' that started radiation and radical prostatectomy on their downward slide. The slide was accelerated by the USPSTF decision on PSA. But it was surveillance that came earlier in 2005-2009 (M. Cooperburg op cit. above) that cut into the numbers. In turn, the sharp rise in surveillance was caused by the first reports of PSA screening studies in 2009 as described in Chapter 3.

I was not cheered by the development of surveillance in Canada or anywhere because it continued the unnecessary biopsy business. It has caused a large number of biopsies, as many as twelve when doing systematic biopsies at a six month interval. Biopsies are still being done in Canada via the transrectal route. The systemic infection rate (some fatal, see Chapter 4) continues at 5% with rising antibiotic resistance. In an earlier publication, Prof. Klotz had reported a 53% radical prostatectomy/radiation for 'cure' rate at five years post the start of surveillance. Fortunately, this high rate of radical surgery following surveillance did not continue.

He presented a moderating factor in his slides at the IPCU 2017 which was improved understanding of the genetic difference between Gleason 3 and Gleason 4. Gleason 3 is not metastatic; it does not have the required genes to do well in bone marrow for example. If all the biopsy shows is Gleason 3 which is not extensive (no Gleason 4), if the magnetic resonance image is not suspicious, and if the PSA density is <1.0, then surveillance is safe. I was disturbed by the MRI he showed us as an example of surveillance. The nodule that lit up was perfectly palpable by the rectal finger at much less expense. In the United States, urologists are now auditing themselves and being audited for 'value.' The federal government will penalize urologists 7% for being more expensive than their colleague for the same clinical result. The MRI discovered nodule is going to lose money to the M.D. who still does the digital rectal exam.

I accosted Prof. Klotz at the bar in the evening of his lecture at IPCU 2017 with my critique which was the high (53%) radical prostatectomy/radiation rate five years post biopsy in an earlier report of his. He reassured me that Canadian urologists in 2017 were responding less drastically to signs of cancer progression than in earlier years. In 2017, at the five year evaluation, Prof. Klotz and his colleagues were agreeing to much less radical surgery and radiation and more focal therapy such as high frequency ultrasound or focal cryosurgery of the nodule under ultrasound control. Better, but not best, in my opinion. The Hopkins group was 'treating' 39% and the UCSF group was treating 40% at the five year evaluation point. We can easily imagine what 'treatment' meant in these two teaching institutions. And so, surveillance in the USA did not mean just that. It meant action 40% of the time.

The cessation of the epidemic depends in the cessation of all biopsies not allowed by PSA modification, palpable target, or increased genetic risk. The biopsy is, in my opinion, "the camel's nose under the tent." And so, I hereby doff my hat to those who are preventing the original biopsy by improved risk stratification.

The chief biopsy preventer in the twenty-first century is E. David Crawford, M.D., Professor of Surgery/Urology/Radiation Oncology, at the University of Colorado, USA. He has organized for many years the annual International Prostate Cancer Update usually in January at Vail, Colorado, but, in 2017 and 2018, at Beaver Creek, Colorado. His paradigm for prostate cancer has evolved drastically in the five years I have been attending his conference.

Most notable is his move past all the various proposed action values for PSA and modifications of PSA (including my beloved density and Proscar suppression) to Select-

MDx, a commercial product that will price at about $500. He dismissed (at IPCU 17) a PSA of 1.5 (ug/ml) in a 38 year old as a surrogate for enlarged prostate (BPH). Hooray! He showed a graph of prostate volume versus serum PSA (ng/ml) is almost a straight line to a PSA of 6.0 at age 65 with 60 cc's of BPH. See Figure 1. The graph was from a famous article by Roehrborn et al in Urology, 1999; 53:581. This was 13 years before the USPSTF pronouncement of 2012. Prof. Crawford published confirmatory data to Roehrborn in 2006. This certainly fit my experience in private practice in the southern San Joaquin Valley of California. I had numerous referrals for an "elevated PSA" in 60 year olds with 60 grams of BPH. 90% of them turned out to be false positives for significant prostate cancer but true positives for significant BPH. I presented this data as a poster at IPCU 2016. Nobody threw bricks at me.

Serum PSA>1.5ng/ml Predicting Enlargement & Risk of Progression of BPH

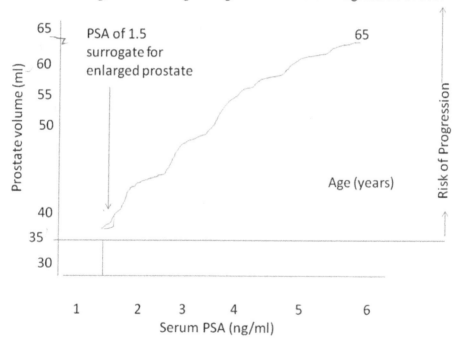

FIGURE 1

It shows that a 65 year old man with 60 ml's of BPH usually has a PSA of 6.0 ng/ml. The mistaken interpretation that a PSA of 6.0, with this much volume of BPH in a man of this age, pointed to significant cancer was one cause of the epidemic of over-diagnosis. (The graph is Prof. Crawford's adaptation of a graph from Roehrborn C.G. et al Urology 1999:53:581-589)

Prof. Crawford does not biopsy all these elevated PSAs. He now demands an 'abnormal' digital rectal exam. This word 'abnormal' has occasioned too many biopsies because

BPH is held by some, not I, to be abnormal. Thirty percent of men develop BPH; an experienced urologist can feel the uniform texture, the symmetry, the lack of invasion of the lateral sulci, and the lack of a rock hard nodule in pure BPH. It may be that the dependence of urologic trainees on the transrectal ultrasound image since 1983, instead of distinguishing between hard and soft that has caused the high frequency of biopsies of BPH, which may or may not be true negatives. Among the positives, Prof. Crawford now calls Gleason 3+3=6 a false positive for significant prostate cancer. The cognoscenti at IPCU now agree with Dr. Klotz of Canada and regard Gleason 6 as lacking the genes to survive as metastases. If mets appear occult Gleason 4 is suspected.

There are now three tests to predict significant prostate cancer with a biopsy, Select-MDx, phi, and 4kscore, each with its proponent on the payroll. Prof. Crawford in the winter of 2017 favored SelectMDx over phi, and 4Kscore. SelectMDx identifies two genes associated with aggressive CaP in urine after a prostatic massage. In the very low risk group identified by the absence of these genes in urine, he has found a 99.6% negative predictive value for Gleason 4+4=8 and 98% negative predictive value for Gleason 7, meaning Gleason 4+3 or 3+4. When these genes, present only in Gleason 4 and above, appear in the urine, we should consider biopsy.

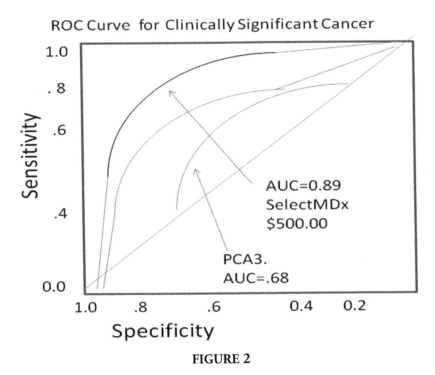

FIGURE 2

The area under the diagonal (AUC) = .5, i.e. half the area of the square. A test with that AUC is as good/bad as flipping a coin. If you want to know whether you have significant prostate cancer, most people would not want to flip a coin. Stand alone PSA with an action value of 4.0 ng/ml has an AUC of about .55 in ages 50-65, i.e. flipping a coin.

The test in Figure 2 was published in European Urology 2016 with authors Van Nestle L. et al, and it featured the first 'area under the curve' for a PSA test greater than 8.0, namely, 8.9. Nobody, in the PSA literature ever says what a good AUC is, probably because for stand alone PSA the AUC = 5.5, flipping a coin. The graph in Figure 2 is entitled ROC (receiver operator characteristics) for clinically significant prostate cancer. The AUC of a competing test, PCPTRC(4K) is an almost good .77, but adds age and digital rectal exam into the mix. The two data points may be contributing most of the specificity. Still another is .68 for the now well known PCA3. SelectMDx shows a significant difference (p>.001) between patients with Gleason scores of 6 or less and 7 or greater. The distinction between Gleason 6 and Gleason 7 makes this test a winner over PHI (a combination of total PSA, free PSA, -2proPSA) which features a large overlap of standard deviations between the two grades, i.e. no significant difference. Dr. Crawford's summary of the good characteristics of the test is that it has 100% sensitivity and 100% negative predictive value if the cut off Gleason score is 4+3 and above and if the clinician uses 3+3 and 3+4 as non-action value. This was his personal series of 73 consecutive private patients in 2018.

I have a quibble with all of this; it is price. SelectMDx comes in at $500. The others are the same except 4K, which is $1900, a preposterous figure. My practice was almost totally Medical-Medicare, much of it in narrow networks of managed care. The managed care plans are not going to pay for these tests. I have used PSA density and Proscar suppression as described in Chapter 1 since 1989 to separate BPH from cancer. None of the tests above have been run against PSA density. Prof. William Catalona admitted in his point counterpoint debate with Prof. Peter Carroll at the 2016 annual meeting of the Western Section of the AUA, that PSA density .15 is an excellent way to find high grade prostate cancer. At the same debate, Peter Carroll said that the digital rectal exam should be brought back to practice because of its excellent specificity! So here we are re-inventing the wheel. I presented a poster to IPCU 16 showing the results of triaging private patients referred for 'elevated PSA' by PSA density and the Proscar suppression test described in Chapter 3. It divided into a BPH group and a suspicion of cancer group. In the latter, it was 91% false positive for significant cancer, i.e. Gleason >6. The BPH group was 90% true positive for BPH. Many of them chose microwave therapy for cure. As modernizing nations begin to catch the PSA 'virus,' I think they should save $500 and biopsy only those with a PSA density >.15 or who do not suppress with three months of finasteride (Proscar) to ½ the presenting 'elevated PSA,' preferably below 4.0 ug/ml. This modification of screening will taper the epidemic measurably.

CHAPTER 19

Whole body, i.e. systemic, therapies are now overtaking those aimed only at the original site of the cancer

The belief that prostate cancer could be 'cured' by its discovery before the development of metastases via radical excision/radiation to the primary site has been withering coincident with the discovery of more effective systemic therapies. They are: (1) early chemotherapy; (2) statins, aspirin, and metformin; (3) immunotherapy; (4) early and more complete gonadotrophin suppression; and (5) a new radiopharmaceutical.

Early chemotherapy, as presented by Daniel Petrylack, M.D., of Yale University, at IPCU 17, means that chemotherapy "now should be considered for patients with extensive disease at the initiation of androgen blockade." He quoted the protocol of the E3805 CHAARTED treatment study. This randomized early docetaxel at 75 mg/m2 every 21 days for 21 days for a maximum of six cycles + androgen deprivation versus androgen deprivation alone. On January 16th, 2014 median follow-up of 29 months, the group reported 136 deaths in androgen deprivation alone versus only 101 deaths when docetaxel, a traditional cell poison, was added to androgen deprivation. The results were most dramatic with high volume disease. There was life extension of 17 months with a near simultaneous collapse after six to seven years. A European trial of the same protocol did not show an advantage for early chemotherapy probably because it was contaminated by too many non-cancer deaths. The E3805 trial was confirmed by another trial called STAMPEDE. You can take this result to the bank.

Similarly the advantages of statins, aspirin, and metformin in prostate cancer as put forth at IPCU 17 by Mark A. Moyad, M.D., M.P.H., Director of Preventive/Complementary and Alternative Medicine, Dept. of Urology, University of Michigan Medical Center, are likewise certain. In Korean, USA, and U.K., he found a 45% reduction in prostate cancer deaths by statin usage after radiation (Park HS et al Ann Oncol 2013) or radical prostatectomy (Song C, et al, Prostate 2015). He found evidence in the literature of multiple mechanisms of cancer inhibition among them, the statins' well known anti-inflammatory properties. The most effective he cited was Rosuvastatin with a 19 hour half-life. The same effect might be achieved by Ezetimibe, a blocker of GI cholesterol absorption.

Prof. Moyad also presented evidence at IPCU 17 that chronic aspirin or NSAID usage reduced prostate cancer by 19% in the REDUCE trial. He quoted the unpublished Aspirin and Physicians Health Study (Allard C B et al J.Clin. Oncol 2016 suppl 2S; abstract 306) as showing an "after diagnosis 27% reduction in mortality from prostate cancer using > three tablets/week." I have no problem with this use for aspirin because I greatly reduced the size of the decidual cell reaction (a benign functioning tumor) to the invading blastocyst by pretreatment with sodium salicylate in the lab rat in 1964. The boss of the lab, an M.D., had said that the decidual cell reaction looked like cancer. He had asked me to look at implantation of the embryo as an inflammatory event. When writing up the experiments in 1970-71, I found numerous references to the anti-tumor growth property of salicylates.

Evidence for a good effect of metformin (called acarbose in Asia) according to Prof. Moyad, is similarly strong. There was a 40% reduction in colonic polyp formation non-diabetics with BMI of 23 (Higurashi T. et al. Lancet Oncol 2016:16:17). While most of the anti-cancer effect has been reported in other cancers, a Swiss group reported in 2014 (Yu et al in Plos One, 9) that at 1000 mg po bid with n=44 there was a 52% prolongation of time to death and a 36% progression rate for 12 weeks in castration resistant prostate cancer. In summarizing this vast literature, Prof. Moyad said that 850 mg po bid was the most common dose; he recommended that it be taken with meals and titrated with regard to weight loss, soft stool and diarrhea; B12 and magnesium deficiency are possible.

Immunotherapy of prostrate cancer is recovering its former place in systemic therapy. In 1976, I published in Conn. Med. an account of my personal case experience with double freeze cryo' of the primary site to relieve bone pain in castration resistant prostate cancer. I was not alone. The Spanish, University of Iowa, and then U.C. San Diego published the relief of bone pain in stage 4 prostate cancer. But the technique died because United States third party insurers were not interested in paying for three months of pain relief.

The most recent approval of immunotherapy has been for Sipuleucel-T, a technique for inspiring cellular immunity to prostatic acid phosphatase, not prostate specific antigen. To gain FDA approval, it caused a median survival benefit of 4.1 months, P=0.017, according to Kantoff et al NEJM 2010. Follow-up studies at lower PSA values showed a median overall survival of 13 months, four times the improvement in months that got the FDA approval according to Raoul S. Concepcion, M.D., F.A.C.S. at IPCU 2017. He summarized the IMPACT date of Schellhammer PF et al, Urology 2013. He also called attention to the work of Drake et al (ASCO GU 2014, Abst. 890) which showed that the percent surviving at 30 months could be as high as 80% compared to 20% of controls if three secondary antigens were recruited in addition to prostatic acid phosphatase. This data placed Sipuleucel-T ahead of Docetaxel chemotherapy and ahead of Radium 223 because the oncologist wished to spare the reactivity of the cellular immune system. Also, there are trials being set up to combine Sipuleucel-T with the new total androgen blockade drugs described below.

Prof. Concepcion also reported the remarkable work of Kantoff et al (J. Clin. Oncology, March 2010) that showed in a phase 2 study an 8.5 months improvement in overall survival for PROSTVAC, a recombinant vaccine containing a gene for a tumor associated antigen + with genes for three costimulatory molecules," inside an attenuated fowl pox viral vector. A phase 3 study has been approved by the FDA.

Another attack is immune check point inhibition after cell injury. These have proven effective in the immune-reactive tumors like malignant melanoma. Autoimmune disease, such as ulcerative colitis, is a forbidding side effect. It becomes the 'effect' of treatment. A phase 3 study of Ipilimumab and post-Docetaxel for androgen deprivation resistant cancer has been presented (Gerritsen et al, European Cancer Congress 2013, Amsterdam, abstract 2850). There was only a 1.2 month overall survival, a small difference at a high price. But, there was an eight month improvement in overall survival in those without visceral metastases compared to those with visceral metastases. This was encouraging but has not led to FDA approval (meaning U.S. Medicare will pay) of Ipilimumab protocols. Many protocols for combinations with other therapies are ongoing.

None of this is a surprise to me. In 1973, as I was leaving my urology residency at Columbia-Presbyterian Hospital, I wrote a grant request to the New York Cancer Research Institute, a non-governmental organization focused on the immunotherapy of cancer. It was run by the daughter of a head and neck surgeon, William B. Colley, based at New York's Memorial. It specialized then and now in the immunotherapy of cancer. Around 1905, this New York head and neck surgeon had a patient with a sarcoma of the neck that got infected with streptococcus, a.k.a. erysipelas, and then it melted away. W.B. Colley then invented a vaccine made of mixed streptococcal toxins that he inoculated into sarcomas in his practice. Some of them melted away. My grandfather, John Rogers Jr., M.D., on staff at Memorial, treated two sarcomas this way about 1905 and published them. I read the two papers in 2016 on the internet, courtesy of the New York Academy of Medicine. One patient had the sarcoma wrapped around his spinal cord; he could not walk. The second had the sarcoma wrapped around the hip and couldn't walk. Both walked months after the injection of streptococcal vaccine and seemed to be cured. The tone of the articles by my grandfather was very matter-of-fact. He did not seem surprised.

Alas, my grant request was not funded even though it was based on a widely noted phenomenon, that cryosurgery to the primary site of prostate cancer will, if two sessions are separated by about two weeks, cause the bone pain of prostate cancer to diminish in 30% of patients. It lasts about three months and then has to be repeated. I published the patients I took care of directly in Connecticut Medicine in 1976. My idea was to study the lymphocytes, the T-cells now, to see which patients were anergic. That might explain some of the non-responders. I still think it is a good idea.

Cryosurgery is a natural immune stimulant. The antigenic groups are left intact on the surface of the cancer. Radiation therapy is also attempting to jump on the immune bandwagon via the occasional observation of an abscopal effect; a distant metastasis melts away when the primary site is irradiated. Three groups have demonstrated an immune response in prostate cancer. One used intraprostatic brachytherapy seed placement (Finkelstein et al, 2012), two used external beam to boney lesions + Ipilimumab (Slovin et al, 2013, and Kwon et al, 2014). The best results were by Slovin et al. Eight of 28 had 50% PSA reductions; there was one complete response of >11.3 months. Six of 28 patients had stable disease. These results appear on Raul Concepcion's slides shown at IPCU 17 and give hope for better palliation.

Improved results for systemic androgen deprivation therapy continue to be published. Degarelix, a gonadotrophic-releasing hormone antagonist, had 2% better overall survival than older luteinizing hormone agonists (Miller K. et al, EAU 2013, poster 678). This advantage is greater if there is a previous history of cardiovascular disease. Marc B. Garnick of the Harvard Medical School explained at 2018 IPCU that much of the explanation may be that true antagonists do not stimulate the release of FSH as do the agonist-antagonists. FSH encourages dyslipidemia, insulin resistance, and increase in osteocalcin/RANK/TNFa. FSH stimulates the prostate cancer cells that have become immune to hypogonadal state. Some advantage may be caused by differing response of T-cells modulation of collagen deposition.

Enzalutamide, a super flutamide, and the androgen pathway inhibitor, Abiraterone, have been approved by the FDA in the pre-chemotherapy, castration resistant setting. So has Apalutamide, a second, new super-flutamide. The FDA approved it in 2018 because it significantly delays the appearance of visible metastases.

Another source of hope, as mentioned earlier for good palliation, is FDA approved Radium 223. It is an alpha emitter with short range and causes double stranded breaks in the DNA. When paired with a true placebo, it gave 2.6 months extra overall survival. Those with no prior Docetaxel got 4.6 months overall survival. By combining Radium 223 with Denosumab, an anti-osteoporosis medication, the patients got three more months of life (Saas et al, ASCO, 2015). With Radium 223 + Abiraterone, two months of life were gained. Remarkable separation was achieved between one to four injections of Radium 223 and five to six injections, i.e. six months to 18 months (Sartor et al, ESMO/ECCO, abstract 2530). As with all other treatments, the earlier they are started, the more difference they make.

As at IPCU 17, strong evidence was presented by Mark Moyad, M.D., at IPCU 18, that diet and weight training improved prostate cancer survival. He showed slides of the adverse effect of aging on muscle physiology and how aerobic resistance training can fight it. He lectured at IPCU 17 on exercise and dietary supplements. The best reference I could find was not in man, prostate cancer, but in the colon-26 mouse aerobic or resistance training exercise model. Khamoui et al showed that aerobic wheel running, "...may have preserved function, and reduced the inflammatory response of the spleen..." (Metabolism 2016 May; 65(5):685-98); resistance training, not so much.

CHAPTER 20

Coda

"Now integrate!" professorial marks in the margin of my solution to an electricity question in my final exam in Physics 101 at Dartmouth college in 1959.

The professor's words still rankle 43 years later. I had taken an electricity problem halfway, and then failed to use calculus to derive the answer. I will not make the same mistake twice. I will integrate. Here is my synthesis of the plague years. E.O. Wilson would call it consilient science. This synthesis resembles the emerging consensus about the cause of the worldwide credit collapse of 2007-2008. Experts say that the bonds were analyzed closely for risk of failure, but nobody added the risk of systemic failure to their calculations. An irrational, worldwide credit bubble was inflating even in Iceland. Experts say that chaos theory analysis could have prevented the catastrophe which followed, but it was not applied.

A prostate cancer bubble has occurred for the same reasons. To technical developments, like the miniaturization of ultrasound and PSA was added the greatest peacetime expansion of an economy the world has ever known. The bull market caused a federal surplus under President Clinton and temporarily took the cost of the Medicare/Medicaid off the national political agenda. The thirty year bond was going to be retired. The cost of prostate cancer care was hardly noticed by Congress because tax receipts were pouring in. The states could afford the cost of Medicaid. Medicare could afford to pay more than a billion dollars for radical prostatectomies. Just as nobody noticed that the eagles were disappearing from the United States due to DDT, nobody noticed the 2815 excess deaths within thirty days after radical prostatectomy because they were scattered over the entire United States and fourteen years of time. Even less notice was taken of 924 deaths (my estimate) following sepsis after transrectal biopsy and less than that of the 11,000 with urinary incontinence. 450 of them harbored suicidal ideation. Nobody cared at all about the 237,284 persons with unsatisfactory sex lives. Fewer orgasms of

137

lower quality in sixty-year-old women were not good television. Science has trouble recording an absence, a void. There was no advertising revenue in the story.

As documented in Lynn Payer's *Medicine and Culture*, the method of payment for medical care elected by a nation determines what medical care is given. In Belgium, where surgeons are paid by the stitch, it takes many stitches to close a laceration. In Britain, where surgeons are paid by the length of the laceration, not by the number of stitches, fewer stitches seem necessary. Urologic surgeons are salaried and so the fewer operations they do the more they make per operation. Surgery rates are low. As a consequence of this climate of opinion regarding all surgery, fewer British than American urologists would submit to a radical prostatectomy. Once when I was making rounds with the Oxford University urology service, a British resident whispered to me, "the only operations we do here are emergency procedures on persons with political influence." Payer also showed tellingly how each version of universal insurance arose like a different plant adapted to the differing cultural soils of France, England, Germany, and the United States.

The United States elected, because of its libertarian character, a system for payment in Medicare/Medicaid that is not a system at all. It is more like Lindblom's business as a form of government. It is a government-subsidized, fee-for-service, price-controlled market. In 1965, Medicare's first year, Congress said that the government would pay "usual and customary fees" for "reasonable and necessary" encounters and treatments for citizens of 65 or over. This bizarrely broad coverage resulted from a Republican fear of being left behind in a Democratic push to pass a bill that paid for hospitalization. The Democratic version of the bill had a deductible that would put the brakes on spending, the doctor's fee. The Republican version of the bill paid for doctors, but left the far larger hospital charges as the deductible. Either of these two out-of-pocket costs would have been the fiscal brakes. But when it became clear to the Republicans that the Democrats had the votes to pass their hospital bill, the Republicans tacked on their doctor's bill insurance to get some of the political credit for something that was going to happen anyway. The Office of Management and Budget did one overnight computer run to test the effect of cobbling the two bills together. The bill passed the next day. And so we had and have a program with virtually no brakes on spending. It was totally irresponsible of Congress to pass it. As a practical matter, if there is a code number to represent an operation in the Medicare carriers' computers, surgeons will do it and patients will ask for it. There has always been a code number for radical prostatectomy and radiation.

By way of illustration of how the United States business-as-government scheme works, consider the case of cryosurgery for prostate cancer. I was paid in my private practice days in the 1970s for cryosurgery of the prostate for palliation of late stage bulky bleeding cancer. This had the happy effect of relieving the bone pain in about one third of the cases through a presumed immune effect similar to the Dendreon product.[471] In one patient, I was able to freeze the cancer wrapped around his ureters and so unblock his kidneys. He died free of pain with normal renal function; no tubes either in his urethra or sticking out of his sides. It was a good death. The same code I used in the 1970s for this man, was used, in the 1990s, for cryosurgery for putative cure of incidental and occult cancer at the time of discovery. This became a default practice for persons who refused radical surgery. For two years, Medicare showed some moxie and denied payment for this use of the code so early in the disease. Cryosurgery sold as a cure disappeared from practice. Surveillance, meaning no treatment at all, increased. Nobody commented because science has trouble recording zero.

Finally, after several papers showed destruction of cancer cells in the prostate in a short time frame, Medicare relented and began to pay for the code again. Cryosurgery again took off in terms of utilization, absolute numbers of procedures. The zero rate of surgery during the denial period proved that the citizens, not yet suffering patients, were not willing to pay out of pocket to save their lives. Alternatively, the patients kicked the tires of cryosugery and found them too soft to warrant out of pocket expense. Once Medicare started paying again for the procedure, United States urologists had no trouble obtaining consent from the citizens for cryosurgery with a pretense of cure. This proves to me that prostate cancer care depends on the profit to the medical-industrial complex.

The definition of the words "reasonable and necessary" in the 1965 Medicare legislation was not tackled by the Medicare carriers until April, 1999. There is still no statement about the relation of aggregate cost to the federal budget of all the listed diagnosis-procedure-code pairs. Only in April of 1999, thirty-three years after the legislation, did Medicare publish a notice in the Federal Register about the process, the steps to be followed by the Medicare carrier, in the determination of what services are covered in the case of what diagnosis.[472] Workers for Medicare carriers are forbidden to give out to M.D.s diagnosis-procedure pairs that are payable. They can only direct the doc to a website where payable pairs are listed. Their claim that to give out payable pairs would be to give advice is spurious. Notice of what pairs are payable does not constitute advice to use those pairs in a particular clinical situation. If we docs use the wrong pairs, we are liable for recovery with penalties in the event of an audit. The professional onus to code correctly is on us, not the Medicare carrier, just as members of Congress have an obligation to report their travel expenses accurately for reimbursement.

Only a few urologists in the world were holdouts from the bubble of care excited in the poorly conceived Medicare/Medicaid in the United States. The British have been notable dissenters. The British elected capitation for general practice after World War II. This meant a generalist was paid the same fee for a person, sick or well, for a year. Specialists and surgeons were salaried in hospitals. Under this Skinnerian schedule of rewards and punishments, the members of the British Association of Urological Surgeons Working Party on the Diagnosis and Management of Early Prostate Cancer wrote in 1999 that "…the apparent reduction in mortality and prolonged survival times with increased case finding are to be expected as a result of lead time and length bias."[473] They did not buy into radical prostatectomy. They went on to say, "Even in the best departments, positive margin rates are obtained which would be unacceptable in other tumor types."[474]

But their position paper was not flawless. They stated, for example, that "radical prostatectomy is the only treatment which accurately defines the true disease stage."[475] This says that you have to have the prostate and its adjacent tissues in the 'bucket' to know where you are in the natural history of this citizen's disease. This is not true as the earlier chapter on bone marrow aspiration attests. The working party went on to write that "...radical prostatectomy, correctly performed, will eradicate the disease if it is confined to the prostate...." Here they lapsed into a tautology. Tautology is content free like giving the baseball scores, but not who won and lost. This sentence says that the operation eradicates all the disease if it eradicates all the disease. To escape this tautology, a statement is needed as to whether this cancer is confined to the prostate at the time the operation typically is done. The reader now knows that it is not. The British Working Party sensed their tautology when they discussed removing the radical prostatectomy from the list of approved operations in the national health system. They rejected the idea on the grounds that Britain is a democracy and the voters would have rebelled.[476]

Let us go deeper. The Walsh-British tautology above is the pinched legacy of David Hume, a Scottish philosopher active in the early nineteenth century mentioned earlier. The quotation usually cited to outline his position is this:

"Let the course of things be allowed hitherto ever so regular; that alone, without some new argument or inference, proves not that, for the future, it will continue to do so. In vain do you pretend to have learned the nature of bodies from your past experience. Their secret nature, and consequently all their effects and influence, may change, without any change in their sensible qualities. This happens sometimes, and with regard to some objects: Why may it not happen always, and with regard to all objects? What logic, what process of argument secures you against this supposition? My practice, you say, refutes my doubts. But you mistake the purport of my question. As an agent, I am quite satisfied in the point; but as a philosopher, who has some share of curiosity, I will not say skepticism, I want to learn the foundation of this inference."[477]

With Hume's attitude as a philosopher, not "an agent," Congress would never have authorized the money that put a robot on Mars. They would have worried that Newton's formula for the effect of gravitation might be rescinded on launch day. In some sense, Hume was right at the level of subatomic particles. We know their paths as probabilities only. Einstein hated that finding. "God does not roll dice," he said. However, as the quarks, mesons, and muons aggregate into atoms, then compounds, their aggregate behavior becomes ever more certain. So certain that, as I write, we have put a robot on a moon of Saturn, Titan. To spend all this money, we have to trust with Mr. Hume as an "agent" (his word) that the spheres will circle just as they have for quite a while.

Mr. Hume seemed properly rigorous in 1830, a time when superstition governed large parts of the earth including the Celtic edges of the British Isles. In the field of cancer, the Hume as a philosopher argument suggests that, just because everybody with a certain histology on the biopsy developed metastatic disease if they lived thirty years, does not mean this patient here, today, will do the same. The cancer-as-a-business juggernaut has cleaved to Hume the philosopher, and forgotten Hume the "agent." The common man does not understand probabilities or he would never buy lottery tickets. United States citizens are prejudiced in favor of Hume, the philosopher, because his belief in the possible sudden reversal of the laws of nature corresponds to the optimism noted by DeToqueville, our can-do character as contrasted with the fatalism of Europe. Optimists selectively migrated here and then moved West.

In regard to the vexing issue of screening in Britain, the working party said, along with the United States Veterans Administration, "there is insufficient evidence available either to support or deny benefits from diagnostic PSA testing." This is the sound of one hand clapping. This position contrasts with the American and Canadian Urological Associations' support for an annual administration of the PSA test. The Working Party gave almost equal weight to watchful waiting but failed to point out that watchful waiting, when intelligently implemented, assumes early androgen ablation will be the next step.

Some say the evidence that screening is good is that nationally, except for Wyoming, the prostate cancer death rate is coming down. What pro-screeners never say is that the death rate went up dramatically with the introduction of PSA testing in 1986 and that it is coming down from an iatrogenic peak. Radical surgery in the over age 75 group, common from 1987 to 1992, has become rare except here in the southern San Joaquin Valley where one of our office workers lost her father, aged 85, within 30 days of radical prostatectomy. The death peak was caused by postoperative heart attacks and pulmonary emboli in men subjected to radical surgery, not cancer. A descent from that peak is, therefore, not cause for celebration. A second reason for the declining death rate is the fact that the 30 to 60% of radical prostatectomies that were margin positive triggered an enormous, expensive, unmonitored, early androgen ablation practice. Such a practice, while truly extending cancer specific life, may shorten arteriosclerotic specific life.

Ivan Illych was not the first to say[478] that western European doctors caused as much illness as they cured. George Washington and Lord Byron died of bloodletting. Moliere in the seventeenth century and Daumier in the nineteenth got in some pretty good licks. But even they did not say, like Illych, that lay people should become their own doctors. In my view, the laicization of medicine, Illych's cure and French deconstruction's delight, is partly responsible for the prostate cancer care epidemic. The students at the barricades in Paris and some professors here told our citizens that, since language had no fixed meaning and science is impossible, they were equal to the docs. Many fell for the ruse. They were told to choose an option as though they were choosing their supper from a menu. An advertisement for the Theraseed brand of radioactive seeds offered "one happy significant other," a good point regarding quality orgasms on the distaff side, but not true after more than two years follow up, a study that may never be done because of its cost and its probable findings. The advertisement assumes that our citizens are up to the doctor's role; they are consumers strolling in a medical Walmart.

The vast cognitive asymmetry between the citizen and the M.D. in this assumption has been ignored. I see this as part of Fukuyama's "great disruption." As part of the disruption, medical students were empowered to choose their own electives as though they knew the relative frequencies and intensities of the diseases they would encounter when licensed. The production of specialists was discouraged and the production of generalists ramped up. The production of midlevel caregivers, nurse practitioners, and physician assistants, was also increased. "Between 1987 and 1997, the proportion of patients who saw non-physician clinicians rose from 30.6% to 36.1%. There was an increase in the proportion of patients obtaining preventive services from non-physician clinicians."[479] Psychologists clamored for and obtained in some states the drug prescribing privileges that had been reserved for M.D.s.[480] The presence of an osteopath is required by law on the Medical Board of Wyoming concerned with M.D.s. Optometrists angled for prescription privileges for medications. Only one in sixteen health care workers was an M.D. in the early 1980s as compared to one in three in the early part of the century after Flexner's reforms.[481] Could it be that mid-level clinicians were partly (here I do not want to absolve my M.D. specialty and the radiation oncologists of their guilt) responsible for some of the money that flowed to the manufacturers of the flawed PSA test?

All these interest groups had support from U.S. adherents to French deconstruction. They said that a claim of scientific expertise by a member of the Northeast M.D. community, such as myself, was merely a power play, an attempt to make more money. Many people believed them. The conservative, science oriented Northeast was upstaged by St. Louis, MO, and Fresno, CA, in a medical Jacksonian revolution. Areas with a low or normal density of urologists had the highest frequency of radical prostatectomy. A low density of urologists signals low income, less education. Manhattan and San Francisco, over supplied with urologists, had low rates on high income, well educated men. The epidemic was not democratic at all, both because the educated and rich defended themselves against unproven modalities and because these old rich cities had old universities more committed to science than the more recently founded schools. Out in the boonies, the influence of urologists with focused, extra experience at the bench with whole animals waned.

A gooey kind of California hot tub medicine increased in popularity. Candace Pert, Ph.D., in her splendid book, *Molecules of Emotion*,[482] describes her own personal journey in that direction. So did Max Lerner in his cancer memoir cited earlier. Prof. Pert discovered the endorphin receptor after her thesis advisor told her to drop the project. Later, she used her unflagging American optimism to invent a cancer preventive strategy. It has no numbers to back it up, just intuition. It might or, with equal probability, might not be true.

Within this new found respect for innumerate enthusiasm, the epidemic of radical prostatectomies and radiation flourished. The vast majority of the citizens who were sucked into the epidemic with incidental and occult cancers were not cancer patients, *i.e.* sufferers, unless they chose a treatment that subsequently hurt them. This is why I have used the word, citizen, throughout this book. As part of the often valid critiques of modern, western medicine, made by Professor Pert, Ivan Illych and Max Lerner, our citizens exercised, except for Asians and Hispanics in California, what seemed to them common sense. To hell with the discipline of prospective, randomized, controlled medical trials. To hell even with preliminary trials in laboratory species. They said in effect, "I want you docs to screen for prostate cancer and cut it out or irradiate it if you find it." Forget the cognitive asymmetry between M.D. and the citizens.[483] The cognitive authority of our citizens was their humanity. Medicare, Medicaid, and private insurance had no brief to challenge the general hullabaloo.

In my opinion, our citizens are not sufficiently educated, to make these decisions correctly. My father, a Wall Street lawyer who took chemistry in high school, did not know where his liver was. The "great disruption" generated a lack of respect for western science. Western science was presented by honey-tongued humanists as a result of the patriarchal,[484] northwest European male hunger for hegemony.

The medical-industrial business complex was glad to ignore science. An opportunistic compliance with the ill-considered, innumerate desires of the demos paid the rent. Even in a more socialist democracy, the British Working Party could not bring itself to refuse to pay for radical prostatectomy even though their deliberations led that way. Each supposedly non-profit business unit within the United States understood that yielding to the culture of action, *i.e.* cutting and burning, gave it a return on investment advantage over its numerous competitors. In October 2008, the Weil Cornell Physicians faculty practice plan in New York bought a full page ad in the Sunday *New York Times* magazine extolling Dr. Ashutosh Tewari as the director of robotic prostatectomy. They neglected to say that the operation has not been shown to lengthen cancer specific life. The University of Pittsburgh Hospital's managers have moved into a skyscraper, according to the Wall Street Journal. Thomas Friedman's democratic, free market, entrepreneurial locomotive has rolled along with no one in the cab.[485]

CHAPTER 21

Prescription

Vivere tota vita discendum est- You must learn to live the whole of your life (Seneca)[486] "...Reducing the risk of prostate cancer diagnosis is a clear benefit. It avoids the risk of over treatment (90%), need for surveillance and cancer survivor label with its attendant adverse effect on quality of life.[487]
—Lawrence Klotz, A.U.A. News, 2007

W hat should he/she/we do about the advertisements for prostate cancer screening I saw on New York City subway platforms? What about prevention and various therapies? If pre-cancer is found, 200 mcg/day of L-selenomethionine[488] combined with vitamin E, and lycopenes (raw tomatoes) seemed in the recent past to be able to prevent progression to invasive cancer. It works in rats with precancerous cytology. Vitamin E stopped a human cancer from dissolving an artificially induced basement membrane.[489] But extra selenium and vitamin E have not worked out in man as we have learned from Mark Moyad, M.D., a University of Michigan urologist and our expert on supplements.[490] Genisten, an inhibitor of an enzyme that causes masking and unmasking of cancer causing genes on aging DNA, has reduced "the PSA levels in a majority of men on active surveillance for prostate cancer in a preliminary clinical survey."[491] Soy products when fed to rats prevent the transition from a pre-cancerous state to invasive cancer in an elegant rat model.[492] This seems harmless if not done to excess. In regard to supplements and diet of all kinds, the best synthesis is, according to Dr. Moyad, if it is good for your coronary arteries, it is good for your prostate.

Do not allow a PSA to be drawn without a rectal exam, significant voiding symptoms, and an estimation of the prostate volume. A false positive can make you uninsurable, even unemployed. If the PSA density is <.15 ug/dl/cc prostate, you can turn your attention to more important causes of your coming demise, like accident prevention. More men die of accidents than prostate cancer. For example, I was nearly decapitated in 2006 by a 300-500 pound elk who chose to attempt to leap over my car while

144

I was traveling 60 miles per hour in a snow storm on I-80. I would have looked foolish at my autopsy if I had just had radical prostate surgery. If you have already stumbled into the commercial pit that is modern cancer care and have been told your PSA is elevated, do a 'Proscar test.' Take three months of Proscar 5 mg or Avodart .5mg and then do a PSA. It should be ½ its former value and probably below 4.0. if the BPH is less that 60 grams.

I would wait for a rock hard nodule characteristic of prostate cancer to be found by an experienced urologist before agreeing to a biopsy. That way you weed out the 380 insignificant, occult, incidental cancers that characterize the prostate over 40. It is fairly safe to say that if an experienced urologist does not feel it, it will not overwhelm you if you have less than 30 years life expectancy. Of course, non-specialists and urologists with little experience will feel the hot breath of the lawyers pushing them to declare a suspicious nodule. Even after nearly 40 years experience, 15 in the V.A. system as World War II came through, I have moments of indecision. High grade cancers, 20% of prostate cancer deaths, don't form much of a nodule and are a constant worry.

This biopsy should be transperineal and directed by the rectal finger toward a palpable, suspicious nodule. It should not be occasioned by a so-called elevated PSA. Two passes through the nodule and one to the uninvolved side should suffice. I could do this with local anesthesia in the tough, World War II vets. The pathologists may cry out for more tissue but they do not have to deal with the miserable prostatitis that can follow the fashionable 21 cores obtained in non-sterile fashion via the rectum.

If a significant, meaning middle grade in a large amount or high grade in small amount, cancer is found, what should you decide about the primary site and what about the certainty of metastases? In my opinion, these are not your decisions. I differ with Ivan Illych, Jacques Derrida, and Michael Foucault. I believe he, or the couple, should pay a good doctor without conflict of interest in the results to broker the strident claims of those with conflict of interest.

But who is a good doctor? My model for a good doctor is the late Bradford Walker, M.D., of Cornwall, Connecticut, where my parents had a summer house and where we kids had a few medical events. By the 1970s, Dr. Walker had the oldest, active medical license in Connecticut. It dated from 1923. He faced competition from time to time in his 50 years of practice but nobody came close to dislodging him from the loyalty of the people of Cornwall. He was recruited to the town right out of Yale Medical School, a Flexner favorite, and given a first year income guarantee. My mother believed he had had a residency in ENT and then returned to general practice. Whatever his credentials were, he delivered babies, did tonsils 30 minutes away at the hospital in Torrington, and worried about the people of Cornwall.

I recall him coming by our house after his rounds in Torrington to check me when I was about ten and had a viral pneumonitis. The lung had turned solid and I was pretty sick. He would come sweeping in, somber as a judge at sentencing time. I never saw him smile. He thumped my chest, listened to the lungs, and was gone in an instant. No glad handing. No public relations with us because we were from the city and had money enough for a weekend house. He once told the voluble mother of a summer child like myself, "If you don't stop talking, I won't be able to hear what is wrong with this child," and earned the child's unending gratitude.

When my twin sister cut off the tip of her finger in a lawn mower about age five, Dr. Walker instantly referred her to his son just starting as a general surgeon in nearby Litchfield. He had no ego about such things. Years later, when, as a graduate student at the Harvard School of Education, my sister returned to Dr. Walker to be treated for parasites acquired in India, she also consulted him about her case of hepatitis A. She felt weary and without energy a year after the acute attack. The Harvard Student Health Service had diagnosed her as another anxious graduate student. Dr. Walker said in the low, gruff voice I can hear as I write, "Lib, it takes two years to get over hepatitis." That was all. He had before him a chart that contained some preschool immunizations and the day of the missing finger tip. He knew from this sparse record that she was not a mental case. His dictum had a pronounced healing effect on her. He had been practicing 50 years. He had known her 20 of those years since the lawnmower incident. On his authority, she decided just to wait the symptoms out. She did not think of him as a patriarchal, white male of northwest European descent determined to maintain hegemony for his sex and pale English skin over women, children, and people of color by constructing a fictional time course for hepatitis. Two years later, almost to the day, she felt her pep return.

One more. My brother's tennis partner wrenched his back playing tennis on a Saturday. He tried to tough it out until Monday, but on Sunday morning found he could not. He called Dr. Walker's home where the office and home were one. The doctor's wife said, "Thank goodness you called. By all means, come down." When he arrived, the doctor's wife greeted him at the door saying, "I'm so glad you've come. Brad has been pacing the floor all morning saying, "There must be somebody in this town who needs me!"

That was our doc. He did no public relations. He did not "grow the business" as they say in the business press. He predated the division of labor into specialties and subspecialties characteristic of post-war medicine. His conscience was, therefore, not divided either. It's my guess that Bradford Walker, M.D., would have dismissed the prostate cancer epidemic as the madness of crowds.

So, here is my Bradford Walker, M.D., inspired prescription for a positive biopsy. When I first composed it in early July of 2003, the 74 degree air on the Wyoming overthrust plateau was clear as gin. The twittering birds in the exuberant grass were mad with song. Max Lerner advised, after his extreme but successful experience with two cancers (one of them an endocrine-responsive prostate cancer which presented in his lung!) that we should take extreme care to live every day of our life. Really live. He became a gym rat at 80. Seneca said the same in the quote above. A man previously paralyzed by a bullet and confined to a wheelchair gave the same advice via the press after he survived in his wheelchair the collapse of I-35 into the Mississippi River near Minneapolis/St. Paul.

A low fat diet is a good idea for your prostate as it is for your heart. We have known for years that cancers of all kinds live on fat. It also keeps your arteries open, a far more common cause of death than prostate cancer. I lift weights for 30 minutes a day, if I don't golf (walking, carrying my bag, no carts), play tennis, or cross country ski in the winter. I am only 10% body fat like Michael Jordan and Scotty Pippen in their prime. Eight years ago, I had a CT scan of my abdomen for duodenal obstruction caused by the Giardia parasite acquired from a crystalline mountain spring. The radiologists had difficulty reading it because they need a layer of fat around most Americans' organs as a frame. They were unfamiliar with an American at his fighting weight. Obesity is strongly correlated with all kinds of cancers.

A low fat diet is indirect treatment. In regard to direct treatment we should not lump all prostate cancers together, as Cornelius Ryan and Michael Korda did in their books. My A.M. radio station just carried a story about a movie star having "the cancer." This is ill-educated nonsense. Aristotle was right to tell us that the subdivision of reality into manageable parts is the first job of science. If you do not know the Gleason grade of your disease, you do not have anything to report. With a gene micro-array test for breast cancer, we are getting close to a DNA signature for each cancer. We are not there in prostate cancer, although we are close. Do not allow best to be enemy of the good. For the purposes of the layman, there are two initial subdivisions of cancer in older adults: (1) the genetically uniform rapidly multiplying cancers that are susceptible to chemotherapy (like the acute leukemias) or radiotherapy (like seminoma) and (2) the heterogeneous cancers, meaning there are many different cell types in any tumor nodule. In 100 patients with a positive biopsy, there will be 50 substantially different varieties. Even within a given deposit there will be substantial variations in DNA. Prostate cancer has that kind of heterogeneity.

Within the heterogeneous cancers like prostate cancer, there are three further subgroups for the lay-person's purposes. They are the well, moderately, and poorly differentiated cancers. That's it. That's all the lay person needs to know. The Gleason grades are useful but not so precise that the lay reader must learn them. Pathologists, in an unguarded moment of truth, will say that the Gleason grades break down into the three above. Recall that the Swedish pathologists disagreed about grade 60% of the time in their recently reported series of radical prostatectomies.

Well differentiated prostate cancer takes 25-30 years to kill the host after discovery. It, like all of them, thrives in bone marrow. It does not thrive in lymph nodes. It makes PSA unless it is poorly differentiated. It is largely androgen dependent. Eighty percent of the cells commit suicide when deprived of male hormone. It is not in the least bit susceptible to radiotherapy or chemotherapy because there are not enough cells undergoing mitosis at any one time. When it is discovered by chance, perhaps in the chips produced by a transurethral resection for benign prostatic hypertrophy, surveillance via rectal exam and PSA tests every six months is all that need be done if it is well or moderately differentiated. Doing nothing to the primary site is very hard for Americans. For that reason, in the case of moderately and poorly differentiated histology, I did cryosurgery in a nerve/sphincter sparing way for those who have not had TURPs. I have done it with no physiologic losses. Frostbite is selective for cancer and it leaves the chemical groups on the cell surface to inspire the immunity that can occasionally be raised against this cancer.

When and if the PSA doubles within a year, have a bone marrow drawn and stained for cytokeratin-16 and monoclonal antibodies against PSA. If it shows positive, lower the male hormone for one and a half years. That encompasses the 475 day doubling time of this cancer. After that, all the cells that are going to die for lack of testosterone have died. The Vancouver B.C. group has shown that intermittent androgen deprivation is as good as continuous in man and animal. You can have your testosterone back. You, your bones, and your wife will notice it.

How to lower the male hormone is a vexed topic because of the high cost of the LHRF antagonist/agonists that arose from Schally and Guillemin's Nobel-worthy experiments. It is enough to say that all methods should be medical. Surgical castration, while clearly more economical, is a grevious psychological hit according to Max Lerner. I have told the reader of the vet who blew his brains out on the ward at Walla Walla the morning after his surgical castration. Agents, such as flutamide, which block androgen action at the peripheral cells, rather than prevent the release of the androgen cascade centrally, are preferable if you want to maintain your sex life. Early peripheral blockade has been shown to delay PSA recurrence. A super cheap method is the old-fashioned one milligram of diethylstilbesterol plus a tablet of aspirin. Anatole Broyard claimed his sex life continued on this pill. This is not for people with a history of risk factors for heart attacks or clots in their legs.

The latest addition to the LHRF antagonists is Degarelix (Firmagon commercially), a pure antagonist. It is FDA approved and produces a crash in the testosterone without causing a flare of testosterone release like the agonist-antagonists drugs Lupron and Zoladex. To antagonize the flare, it is necessary to administer a second drug, Flutamide, that costs $500.00 for a month. This drug has caused bone marrow depression of white blood cells[493] and/or occasional liver failure. Five hundred dollars is too much for my elderly underinsured. Casodex is better in this class. You should time the period of hypogonadism with your activities because it will cut your recall for random words in half, but it will improve your executive ability, i.e. your ability to think about the future. I postponed the treatment for one of my V.A. patients until, at seventy-eight, he had finished renovating his house. He said he lacked initiative as it was. I said, "Okay, finish your house first." Androgen deprivation does not have to be continuous. Intermittent deprivation has the same effect as continuous.[494]

At the time androgens are lowered, your oncologist should consider coincident mitoxanterone, docetaxel, or whatever else is current therapy. The mitoxanterone has been shown by Wang of England to prolong life significantly at ten years in a randomized, prospective, controlled trial. Docetaxels gets you two more months on this earth. It is a microtubule inhibitor derived from the yew tree. More about these poisons in a minute. The lowering of testosterone actually induces the activity of the anti-cell suicide gene for clusterin.[495] Androgen ablation is, in that sense, carcinogenic. You get nothing for free in biology. That is why it is good to hit the cells at the same time from a different angle while they are trying to reorganize to make clusterin. Clusterin confers immortality on the cancer cell. Simultaneous docetaxel and androgen deprivation were on the menu at Memorial Sloan-Kettering in New York in 2007,[496] not early enough in my opinion. Remember that triple drug therapy was found to be necessary in tuberculosis. The first drug discovered to be effective, streptomycin, produced only temporary remissions because it induced resistance. A second and third drug with different mechanism of action simultaneously proved necessary.

When you are undergoing androgen deprivation therapy, you should take a diphosphonate to prevent osteoporosis. An added advantage is that drugs in this class have a direct action on the cancer. In a series of patients in Britain, sodium clondronate had lowered PSA levels and patients were less likely to die from prostate cancer than those not taking the drug."[497] In addition, you probably should take a drug in the cox-2 inhibitor class if you do not have extensive arteriosclerosis. Celebrex is the most commonly known. These sharply focused aspirin look-alikes prevent new blood vessel formation and have been proven to prevent precancerous polyps in the colon. Sketchy reports about improving life span in prostate cancer in man with the aspirin group (NSAIDS) have appeared. It works well in animals. I say this not because I have read it in a book, but rather because I did the following experiment while on a research elective in medical school.

Prof. M.C. Shellesnyak, M.D., Columbia P&S '42 had noted histologic studies that depicted a vigorous infiltration of white blood cells occurred in the lining of the uterus in the first hours preceeding implantation of the invading blastocyst, the fertilized egg. Then, explosive growth of the decidual cell reaction followed. The resultant mass in the uterus was called the deciduoma and it greeted the invading blastocyst at discreet intervals along the tube-like rat uterus.

I began to read the literature about inflammation caused by any non-specific injury, and I came upon some experiments regarding the trauma of turpentine instilled in a rat's pleural space published in 1949 by Spector and Willoughby, two British pathologists. They showed that plain old aspirin plus an antihistamine could profoundly decrease the amount of protein rich water caused by the presence of granulocytes that is to be found with a peak at four hours around any area of injury, *e.g.* a sprained ankle. I thought I would try to stop the swelling and inflammation that precedes ovum implantation with aspirin and then add an antihistamine later in a second experiment.

This spot of inflammation which provides the nest for the invading blastocyst had been earlier identified by Psychoyos, a French investigator. He injected the animals with a blue dye that attached to the large protein molecules in the blood. The implantation sites appeared as intensely blue spots at intervals along the double uterus in the evening of day four after fertilization. This protein-rich blue exudate was not ascribable to histamine. Prof. Shellesnyak thought it was. If I blocked the formation of the exudates with aspirin, the whole laboratory was 'barking up the wrong tree' and Prof. Shellesnyak's job was threatened.

In the rat, the blastocysts implant beginning at seven o'clock in the evening of the fourth day after mating. I was, therefore, alone in a darkened, silent lab. I had pretreated the rats with aspirin every six hours starting at noon of day three. When I opened the first rat there was no blue spot. My pulse raced. I sweated in the cool winter evening. My hands trembled as I opened a control rat not treated with aspirin. There were lots of intensely blue spots evenly spaced. I opened another aspirin-treated rat. No spots. Nine out of nine experimental animals were missing the blue spots. Seven out of seven controls had blue spots. This was a shocking finding; it meant that the professor was wrong and pointed to an entirely new method of birth control as Paul Ehrlich, author of *The Population Bomb*, and the Rockefeller Foundation that funded the lab, would wish.

When I finished, it was four in the morning. I was flooded with catecholamines, the fight or flight molecules. I knew sleep would be impossible. I decided to bicycle to the Mediterranean to try to calm down. I was in Rehoveth, Israel, before the Six Day War. In those days, a tongue of the African veldt extended up between Rehovoth and the sea. An antelope leapt up in the air as I bicycled by him in the darkness. He was as jumpy as I was. The sun came up at my back just as I came to Homer's "wine dark sea." I was reminded of the Phoenicians, later to become Carthaginians, and all the adventurers who had lived on this "old clay where nobody has had therapy."[498] Their tels, ruined cities, were everywhere, bumps on a war ravaged land. In the next weeks, I worked night and day, holidays and weekends, to repeat the experiment and to show that uterine weight was decreased on day seven of pregnancy. They were definitely lighter than controls because the deciduomata were much smaller. Aspirin had caused them to be smaller. I published these findings in a peer reviewed journal six years later.[499]

I tell you, the reader, this autobiography so that you might know the provenance of my confidence. First, that this class of drugs, the NSAID class, will lengthen life in prostate cancer. I have been right as rain in the lab. I do not worry overmuch about pushing back against the entire culture as an experienced clinician after having destroyed the *raison d'etre* of an entire lab funded by the Population Council of New York as a medical student.

This class of drugs, the NSAIDS, is not just 'candy' for joints. They should be medically supervised because they can give you heart attack, renal failure and ulcers. Also, we need the prostaglandins whose synthesis they diminish to dilate our arteries, the coronaries in particular. Take this class if you can while you await approval of other anti-angioneogenetic drugs like Sundilac and Linomide. Avastatin has been approved as has Martha Stewart's drug for colon cancer. The New York Times was right to trumpet on June 6, 2004, "Drugs may turn cancer into a manageable disease."[500] Prostate cancer will be slowed by the NSAIDS as well as by the more precise drugs that target enzymes that are overactive in certain cancers, not all. Chistopher Evans, M.D., Chairman of Urology at U. C. Davis, California, went deeply into this topic at our Western Section meeting in 2008.

The next jump up in ferocity, moderately differentiated (Gleason 7) prostate cancer takes, on average, 17.5 years plus or minus 1.8 years to kill the host, 12 years if it makes a palpable nodule. Some of it, not all of it, makes PSA. Not so many cells are dependent for immortality on male hormone. Like well differentiated cancer, it is only slightly susceptible to chemotherapy. But if it is well along in its natural history, you probably should have a brief, but safe blast of true chemotherapy. It dedifferentiates (becomes more malignant) when subjected to radiotherapy. Radiotherapy is a bad idea for this grade. It goes to both lymph nodes and bone marrow but thrives in bone marrow. The treatments are the same as above for well differentiated but I would not wait for the PSA to double to start lowering your male hormone for 1.5 years. Take an ultrasound picture of the upper urinary tracts to make sure they are not obstructed low down at the bladder level by the cancer. Unless the PSA is above 20 ug/dl, a radioactive bone scan is not useful at this time.

The mean time to death for poorly differentiated prostate cancer (Gleason 8-10) is 6-7 years. It is much more like the breast or lung cancer that has killed your neighbor or relative. This was what Cornelius Ryan and Anatole Broyard had. It accounts for 40% of prostate cancer specific deaths although it is only 10% of cancers discovered. Unfortunately, it does not make the medical student's classic stony hard nodule with sharp borders. It crawls amongst the normal cells to yield only a subtle extra firmness in the normal-sized gland. It is easily missed amidst large nodules of benign prostatic hypertrophy or the scars of bacterial prostatitis as it was, at first, in C. Ryan's case. The PSA may even be normal because the cells have become so primitive that they no longer make this specialized molecule. People die with normal PSAs with this grade. It thrives more in lymph nodes than bone marrow as it did in Cornelius Ryan's case. On a standard X-ray, it makes holes rather than white spots in the bone. Ryan's histology is given in the book as well differentiated, but he must have had a second, poorly differentiated cancer that was undetected. The average number of genetically different cancers in a radical prostatectomy specimen is four. In Ryan's day, numerous widely dispersed biopsies were not common practice. Now they are and small, young cancers other than the ones we feel become part of the specimen.

Cornelius Ryan died within four years. The fact that his wife's book was widely read may have distorted the layman's sense for the time course of this disease or even that of some urology residents. When I presented a poster about Ryan and the other authors at a Western Section of the A.U.A. meeting, an experienced urologist told me that he had urged the Ryan book on his residents. Anatole Broyard's cancer must also have been dreadfully undifferentiated because he died in less than a year. Again, because his book was widely read by the chattering classes, the lay perception of the disease may have become distorted. Poorly differentiated cancers respond minimally to androgen ablation. They do respond briefly to chemotherapy and radiotherapy because their rapid doubling times mean a larger proportion of their DNA is unwound during mitosis and is therefore vulnerable. I have always felt that early chemotherapy must, in poorly differentiated prostate cancer, prolong life. The best evidence is Wang's evidence in England that this is so. In the early 1990s, his group gave three weeks of chemotherapy at the beginning of androgen ablation for palpable local cancer. Ten years later, they could detect statistically significant life extension. For a long time, I thought I was the only person in the western world to notice their report, but I have since learned that it was widely noticed and has inspired a large number of early chemotherapy efforts not yet reported out. Caveat: It is easy for me as a urologist to talk aggressively about these poisons when I do not have to deal with the occasional death from bone marrow failure. My current oncologist colleagues are reluctant to jump in on a patient whose PSA is falling because of androgen deprivation, not rising. They are not so reluctant after the failure of androgen deprivation to prevent a PSA rise. There have been reports of remarkable results with docetaxel, estramustine, and carboplatin.[501] The chemotherapy scene is improving on a monthly basis.

There are localized treatments being applied to the primary site of prostate cancer of which I approve. One is, as above, cryotherapy, the frostbite mentioned in the first paragraph. It depends on the evolution of cryotherapy from liquid nitrogen, with which I trained at Columbia Presbyterian Hospital's urology program, to the use of liquefied argon in very thin needles. When the cold is taken out beyond the capsule of the gland in pretense of cure, it can cause frostbite of the nerves to the penis and sphincter as mentioned above. This should not be allowed to occur because there is no gain. The metastases in the bone marrow set the time of death, not the primary site. Frostbite does not cause cancer to dedifferentiate or cause cancer in adjacent organs like radiotherapy. Bryan Donnelly of the University of Calagary presented a huge series randomize between radiation and cryosurgery and showed equivalence at the Western Section of the A.U.A meeting in October, 2008. He did not track the dedifferentiation caused by radiation in his series but he referred to another that showed a jump in grade that is bad news for the patient.

High intensity focused ultrasound, really a form of heat, has been championed in Germany and looks reasonable, so long as the adjacent nerves and external sphincter are conserved.[502] I do not favor it because the line between cells dead and alive is jagged and indistinct compared to the frostbite line. Another is injecting the primary cancer with absolute ethanol, pickling it. General surgeons have been treating small liver cancers with absolute ethanol injections under ultrasound or C.T. control. Some urologists have reported good results with ethanol in cases of benign prostatic hypertrophy. This simple, cheap technology has been available for a hundred years. It will surely be reported as effective against the primary site of prostate cancer in the near future. Any of these will do no harm, if executed conservatively without intention to cure, *i.e.* the M.D. keeps the cytolytic modality within the prostatic capsule and away from the nerves and external sphincter. Any of them may, in theory, add 1.5 years of extra life if we assume half the cancer cells are in the prostate. The one that provokes the least inflammation will add the most life. This is cryosurgery.

Radical surgery whether done by robot or man has not improved overall mortality at 12 years of follow up in the Swedish study. The scant 5% advantage in cancer specific mortality that appeared at 12 years disappeared by 15 years of follow up, as you would expect in a disease with a mean time to death of 12 years if palpable. Statistical significance disappeared only for the over 65 group.

The Swedes continue to trumpet radical surgery for the under 65 group. I do not know why. Statistical significance will disappear as they get deeper into the natural history. I think they show significance now because only the surgical group gets really 'early' androgen deprivation which is better than 'later' in laboratory species and man.

None of these methods, including radical prostatectomy, will prevent the complications of obstruction of the ureter, bladder neck, and bleeding from tumor nodules that occur in the final two years in 20% of patients. Of all of them, I favor nerve sparing cryosurgery to the primary site because it conserves the surface chemicals on the cancer cell which may, in rare cases, stimulate immunity. Anti-androgen plus chemotherapy in the taxol group is at last being given for initial treatment in poorly differentiated cancer.[503] This study is unfortunately followed by radical prostatectomy. Two patients had no cancer in the specimen and so for them the operation was without value. As in breast cancer, perhaps the radical surgery component will soon be abandoned for the active component, the systemic therapy.

The most important lesson in regard to therapy is that preached by eighty-year-old Max Lerner and the Roman seer, Seneca. Your job on this planet is to live until you die. That means hang on to your sex life as long as you can. Your wife, as the Theraseed ad correctly asserts, will appreciate it. Professor Lerner became a gym rat at eighty. Give up all your bad habits and adopt a healthy life style. You want to be a "sinking ship with nothing to throw overboard."[504] A recent chairman of Urology at Memorial Sloan-Kettering did this for his colon cancer. He lived years longer than his colleagues expected. It was he who showed that rats with prostate cancer on a low fat diet live much longer than those on a normal fat intake. You must, therefore adopt a low fat diet and probably a soy based supplement containing antioxidants.[505] Another 'lifestyler' George Sheehan, M.D., lived seven years after his boney metastases were documented.[506] His silhouette on the book jacket suggests less than 15% body fat.

Immunity to your own prostate cancer is rare. But there are very occasional reports of spontaneous regression. I saw metastatic prostate cancer completely disappear in one of my patients at the Francis Delafield Hospital in New York after two freeze injuries of the primary separated by two weeks. This is not a large number of persons who will develop immunity; we almost never see the white blood cells responsible for immunity gather around this cancer as we often do in the immunogenic cancers (melanoma, ovarian, and kidney). There are very active efforts toward immunotherapy based on PSA secretion by the cells proceeding towards FDA approval by Dendreon as described in the chapter on business. "Therion Biologics Corp. has initiated a multicenter, randomized, double-blind phase II trial to test the safety and efficacy of Prostvac-VF and an immunotherapy for prostate cancer....which...stabilized PSA levels in 52% of early metastatic prostate cancer patients."[507] The problem with this approach is that the worst kind of prostate cancers, the kind that do most of the killing, have lost the genes to make PSA and so will not be killed by white blood cells sensitized to PSA.

If you are still working, do not tell your co-workers that you have cancer of the prostate. Cornelius Ryan did and it was a big mistake in the case of at least one couple who often asked them to dinner. The couple proved to have secret lunacy regarding cancer and its curability by Laetrile available in Mexico. Prostate cancer is a non-starter at work and socially. They may have it too. They just have not pursued it. If you are 60 years old, 50% of your age-mate competitors have microscopic prostate cancers and they are not telling anybody about it. You may lose your job. If you are self employed, you may lose referrals and receipts. You may lose your insurability and you may have to live for many years with less money.

For a bulky cancer near the end that closes quickly after resection, cryosurgery is better than a transurethral resection. If you are weary of procedures, ask the urologist to put in a suprapubic tube by the atraumatic Seldinger technique. Collect the urine in a leg bag. Radiotherapy at this phase can be very effective against bleeding. It is ineffective against bladder outlet obstruction and ureteral entrapment. I favor cryotherapy first because you cannot do it after radiotherapy. If renal function threatens to go below 25% because of obstruction of the ureters, have double J tubes put in your ureters to keep them open. I have opened one set of ureters with cryosurgery but that is unusual. Or maybe not, depending on the extent of your bone pain. If you are near the end, renal failure (uremia) may be a better way to die. You need to write a medical power of attorney before you get to this stage because when your ureters are blocked, your thinking is not clear. You need a will for the same reason. If you are reading this book, you need a recently revised will, not a will you wrote when you were married. I have actually done this.

If bladder outflow obstruction is caused mainly by cancer, not coincident BPH, transurethral resection does not work well. Cancer cell suicide is discouraged by the postoperative inflammation caused by transurethral resection with electrocautery. If it is BPH stiffened and made more significant by the cancer, then a transurethral resection may work better. For a bulky cancer near the end that quickly closes after a resection, cryosurgery is better but Medicare does not pay for it. Ask the urologist to put a tube in the bladder over the pubic bone by the atraumatic Seldinger technique and use a leg bag. Radiotherapy might open it up, if the cancer is poorly differentiated and radiation has not been previously applied.

The final year is characterized by bone pain in most cases. If the cancer in the marrow stimulates the production of bone around it, showing up as white spots on a conventional x-ray, radium-223 (an alpha emitter) given I.V. will localize around the deposits. Of the two patients I contributed from the Walla Walla V.A. to the study of Strontium-89, an older beta emitter, one had magical relief of pain. Strontium-89 can fry your marrow. Radium-223 will be much better because the alpha particle travels a very short distance. It has been shown to lengthen cancer specific life. Two additional drugs for metastases were approved in 2011, with many more to come in the next decade. Now the action turns to the definition of metastasis. Perhaps the criteria should be a PSA above forty and/or cytokeratin positive cells found in the marrow (Immunicon of Hungtington PA).

Narcotics for bone pain at this stage should be prescribed by a pain specialist. But these narcotics are another reason you should have a medical power of attorney and a will already written. Once you are on narcotics, you are not smart enough to handle your own affairs.

Look, this book is an attempt at the generation of wisdom. I had to be hit by an avalanche on Mt. McKinley and hang upside down in the dark in a crevasse at age 27 to learn I was mortal. Surgeons, commodities traders, and senators are optimists, sometimes to the point of delusion. I hope the reader is not delusional. He or she is surely older than I was when hit by an icefall.

There is a banal route to immortality. Hold onto your green eye-shade! It is life insurance and disability insurance. Recent Dartmouth graduates circled my fraternity near my graduation time to sell me insurance as though I were already a corpse on the Serengeti plain. In my youthful wisdom, I ignored them. I ignored the Air Force non-com's counsel that I buy cheap life insurance as part of my mustering out from active duty as an officer. Mistake. I bought my first life insurance and disability insurance after my wife at the time totaled her car on the Henry Hudson Parkway in N.Y.C. She was disabled for full-time work for two years by a head injury. I became enlightened just as Samuel Jackson's character in the movie, Pulp Fiction, was enlightened by a bullet which bypassed his head and lodged in the ceiling. He said it was a sign. Not one of my humanists said a word in their books about their life or disability insurance status. Insurance extends your financial reach beyond the grave. The second time I bought life insurance, at age 49, I had a new wife and a new born son to add to a son by a previous marriage. Both deserved Ivy League educations. On the first, one medical school tuition debt is still pending. If I am killed on CA-99, the most dangerous road in the United States, there is enough insurance to render them debt free. My second wife, who sacrificed ten years of her working life to raise the second child, will not live in penury. I do not, therefore, dissipate my energies worrying about what incidental, microscopic cancers I might have either in my thyroid, or my prostate. I do avoid accidents.

If the reader does not have any or enough insurance, acquire some before you have a PSA drawn and before a biopsy. If the insurance exam requires a PSA, find another insurer. It is not a good test for prostate cancer. Life and disability insurance are far more rational responses to your natural desire for immortality than having a urologist stick your prostate twenty one times[508] with a needle contaminated with feces in an attempt to find an occult, incidental cancer at the edge of an ocean of benign prostatic hypertrophy. Banal as it is, insurance not tied to employment will ameliorate the practical consequences of the remaining 96.4 % of causes of death in men as well as the 3.6 % of prostate cancer deaths. It is the surest way to follow Dylan Thomas's exhortation to "…rage, rage at the dying of the light."

CHAPTER 22

A Glossary of Terms

ADVANTAGES OF THE PLAIN MEANING RULE "The great advantage of the plain meaning rule is that, in theory at least, it creates a zone of certainty — an interpretation-free zone, in effect. It tells the public that if the text is plain, it means what it says and it is safe to rely on it. The courts won't come along and trick you at the last minute by importing unsuspected qualifications or implications into the text, even if these qualifications or implications were probably intended by the legislature. This emphasis on text at the expense of intention ensures that the law is certain and that the public has fair notice, both of which are prerequisites for effective law." Ruth Sullivan, Prof. of Law at the University of Ottowa, in Legal Drafting[509]

T his book will adopt the plain meaning rule as defined above. To read this book you will have to learn some vocabulary.

(1) The word cure: The dictionary gives several definitions, all of which state that the condition is never going to recur. This is the plain meaning as used by lawyers. This is not the meaning given to the word in the prostate cancer literature in the last 20 years. For example, Thomas Stamey, M.D., when still chairman and professor of Urology at Stanford, responded to my questioning him[510] on the meaning of the word by saying he meant 10 years without biochemical (PSA) evidence of recurrence in the blood. Others say 15 years. This modification constitutes the importation of "**unsuspected** qualifications or implications into the text." It is not the plain meaning of the word, *i.e.* the disease will not be evident no matter how long the patient lives. It is a bizarre meaning in the context of prostate cancer because 10 years is not halfway to the median time to death of PSA discovered cancer, 22 years.

(2) 'Controls': The first prospective,[511] randomized,[512] *controlled* study of a medical treatment was published in my life time. It compared streptomycin to no treatment of tuberculosis in 1948. I actually attended a patient at the Walla Walla, WA., Veterans Administration Hospital who was in this original study. He was sent there to die but

joined the study on the streptomycin side and lived instead to a great age to his everlasting satisfaction. Streptomycin proved in his case to be better than nothing. For this outcome to be science, the untreated controls have to be the same age, sex, and health status. The first results of a prospective, randomized, controlled study of radical versus limited surgery for prostate cancer were not reported until 1979,[513] 31 years after the streptomycin trial, and six years after I left my chief residency at Columbia Presbyterian in New York.

(3) Lead-time-bias a.k.a. stage migration: this refers to the fact that, if you discover a cancer earlier in its undisturbed history than heretofore reported the patient will appear to live longer from the time of discovery. This effect is touted by the American Cancer Society as an improved five-year survival rate. It is folly. To clarify by metaphor, it is as if a novel of 300 pages has been opened at the 150 page mark instead of the 250 page mark. The reader appears to have gained 100 pages of reading for his money. In reality, it is the same novel, with the same ending, with the same number of pages. Our citizens know they have a cancer longer. This is why critics of the United States cancer industry demand an improvement in the overall death rate per 100/000. This gives the length of the novel irrespective of where it is opened.

(4) Critics, such as myself, of the cancer business require that a proposed treatment improve the '**death from all causes**' figure rather than the cancer specific death rate. This is because death from cancer usually occurs in an elderly population coincident with other causes of mortality. The cause of death is often not one thing. Another is that it is extremely easy for bias to enter into what is written on the death certificate. In a hospital with a resident training program, the lowest M.D. on the 'totem pole' fills out and signs the death certificate. It is a moment of extreme informality. The institution loses all interest in a patient once he/she has become a corpse. An intern, such as myself years ago, has half a dozen pages on his beeper from R.N.s concerned with the living who do not wish to make a similar transition. Scientific precision in assigning the relative position of the three (only three!- often there are many) causes of death permitted by the form is the last consideration. Protection of senior attending physicians (who may write the intern's next letter of recommendation) from lawyers is the first order of business. Bias in favor of treatments that bring in the money to the hospital to pay his salary is second. If the patient had such a remunerative treatment for cancer, death will tend to be ascribed to the infirmities of old age, not the cancer and certainly not the treatment itself. Conversely, the cancer in the control group, the group not given the proposed money yielding treatment, will tend to be found by the intern (again seeking job security to pay off his student loans) to deserve first place on three cause of death lines on the death certificate. This is one reason why drastic treatments for cancer when remunerative for the hospital and faculty practice plans tend to show an advantage in the cancer specific death rate over less drastic treatments.

An analogy might be Enron's practice of booking a loan as income and hiding the debt in off-shore shell corporations. This did not prevent bankruptcy. It was robbing Peter to pay Paul. It is the same in cancer studies. The robbery of Peter, the misassignment of a cancer death to another cause, *e.g.* cardiac, shows up as a lack of improvement in death-all-causes when the books are reconciled. The 12 year results of the Swedish study of radical prostatectomy versus nothing show no difference in death-all-causes.

(5) Publication bias is another concept poorly understood both by the public and by M.D.s who have not published in peer reviewed journals, which is most of them. Publication of even a simple original article, in my experience, costs about $2,500 in labor. This leads to a vast sea of projects not undertaken or, if undertaken, unpublished. It takes an ear attached to a critical brain that has published to hear the silence surrounding a gap in a data set. It is the sound of nothing. This is why the current rage for evidence based medicine, meaning published, randomized, controlled, clinical series in man, is naïve. Evidence based medicine highlights data which causes profits for some provider, hospital, or some drug/device manufacturer. Otherwise it would not be published and not considered evidence. It is lauded at the expense of attention to unpublished potential studies in human or animal models with implications that might diminish the cash flow to somebody.

Harold Varmus, M.D., former chief of the N.I.H. and a Nobel prize winner, has started an on-line peer reviewed journal of biologic science to address the problem. The price to the author of publication of a peer reviewed journal article consisting solely of re-arranged atoms and electrons whizzing through the air, is going to be about $1500. Right away the public should smell a rat. Where is that $1500 going to come from? We have long passed the stage of gentleman scientists like Benjamin Franklin who used his business wealth to subsidize and publicize his scientific experiments. Let's face it, an M.D. researcher-teacher-clinician is only going to hand over $1500 to Dr. Varmus if he thinks he is going to get it back in increased patient referrals and subsequent fees to support his salary after the money has been laundered by the dean's office.

Here is the iron law of medical science publishing. If the observation of certain phenomena will decrease income for the faculty practice plan or hospital, the research protocol will not be written; if it is written, it will not be funded; if it is funded, the abstract detailing the unprofitable results will not be written; if it is written, it will not be accepted at the annual meeting of its appropriate scientific society. If it is accepted, it will not be for podium presentation; it will be for a poster. If it is a poster; it will be for the session that begins at 7 a.m. or for a non-clinical research session separated from the main action of the meeting. This implies it is not ready for prime time, code phrase for we cannot make more money from this one.

If by chance the poster gets in, the assistant professor M.D. will receive no encouragement from his department chairman to convert it into a journal article. If, in spite of no encouragement, he still writes the article, the work of a week or two in the evenings, it will be sent to referees who stand to lose money if it sees the light of day. Their criticisms will be harsh. The editor of the journal almost inevitably accepts the criticisms of those with this kind of conflict of interest as 'gospel' and rejects the paper. He earns his living the way they do. The paper goes into the suspense file of the author for later revision. But, that day never comes because the assistant professor receives positive reinforcement from his chairman (who controls his salary and recommendations for tenure) for other work that promises to increase the income of the hospital and/or faculty practice plan. His very few spare minutes for research are consumed by the new project since he/she wants tenure (who wouldn't?) and tenure requires publication of articles.

Suppose the paper is published? Well then, it is not quoted. If it is quoted, it is not acted upon except rarely by those who are willing to "blow against the wind." Those M.D.s always pay a price like Semmelweis, an Austrian physician who advocated the washing of hands between examinations of different women in the throws of childbirth. The managed care plans eagerly courted by 'University' hospitals linked to medical schools (and an army of tort lawyers) reward average performance called the 'standard of care,' not above average performance.

As a remedy for publication bias, I envision in some "brave, new world" a virtual, shadow journal for Harold Varmus's creation. It would be called The Virtual Journal of Complications, Negative Results, Unwritten or Abandoned Protocols, and Rejected Papers or VJCNRUAPRP for short. The M.D. would not pay, but be paid $1500 (by whom?) to report complications, negative results, and treatments with expired or unobtainable patents. In prostate cancer studies, the reader will learn the importance of doing nothing. Who in the medical-industrial complex will make more money if no case finding and no treatment is recommended for the citizen? Where does even Harold Varmus's $1500 come from?

The news about publication bias is not all bad. Once in a while, commercially undesirable results will poke through the pile of money that is the price of entrance. This happens most commonly under socialism, *e.g.* when the British Journal of Urology International published my study of the mean time to death in prostate cancer at the V.A. in Fresno. This is a rare event in English-Dutch capitalism. I could afford to hammer away at it because I was on a federal salary at the time.

(6) Options is a technical word, a term of art, in the health policy literature. Here is its use in a sentence from an American Urological Association white paper:

"A policy is considered an option if the health and economic outcomes are not sufficiently well known to permit meaningful decisions...."[514]

I translate the word, meaningful, to mean rational or scientific. I translate the whole sentence to mean that an option is a current treatment that lacks scientific evidence in man or animal that it will do the citizen any good. This word, options, is all through the prostate cancer literature. It reflects the physician as dumb waiter mentality, a waiter who can cook and who knows the menu really well. Imagine your surprise if, upon entering the hospital for pneumonia, your doctor offered you a selection of antibiotics and asked you to chose one as an option. That would put you on your guard, would it not? In my view, it would be a signal that none of the remedies would predictably improve your condition. It is the same with cancer therapy. When you see/hear the word, options, science is on vacation. The New York Times has twice reported that the modern patient is tortured by his new found freedom to choose his/her cancer therapy. Later chapters will show that the modern citizen with a naïve optimism based on an inadequate education in biology tends to choose that which is most remunerative to the medical industrial complex. This is no surprise; the docs emphasize what will pay their rent.

(7) 'Sensitivity' and 'specificity' are technical terms, terms of art, in our literature. Thomas Stamey, retired chairman and still professor of Urology at Stanford, has written, "Sensitivity implies that you know who has prostate cancer and specificity that you know who does not have prostate cancer before applying diagnostic or even biopsy tools, conditions that are clearly never met with prostate cancer."[515,516] More precisely, "sensitivity is defined as the true positive rate, the proportion of those with the disease (as defined by the gold standard) who test positive when the defined discriminant criteria and positivity criteria are used...Specificity is one minus the false positive rate, where the false positive rate is defined as the proportion of those without the disease who test positive."[517] Bayes' theorem[518] says that the trade off between these two characteristics of any test is dependent (this is huge) on an *established prior probability* of a certain result. Thus, prejudice determines the interpretation (not the result) of test. In the case of prostate cancer, only 3.6% of men have a tumor clinically **significant** enough to kill them. With such a low **prior probability** of a significant cancer, Bayesians insist that a useful screening test for prostate cancer must have a high specificity,[519] *i.e.* over .8, or only 20% false positives. Chapter 4 will point out that what we have with the famous PSA test is not 20% but 70% false positives in routine clinical work. We have a specificity of .3, an immense drain on the economy and a source of great misery and the cause for much of this book. See Chapter 4.

The concepts above will be used repeatedly in the book. Putting them here allows the narrative to flow better. The reader must walk before he runs in a market with signs to guide you to a bad place.

REFERENCES

[3]Nutthal A.D. Why scholarship matters. The Wilson Quarterly. Autumn 2003, p. 60, passim.

[4]www.asri.edu/bfisher/press_release2.html.

[5]Smith I.E. and Dowsett M. Aromatase inhibitors in breast cancer.N.Eng. J. Med. 348: p. 24, 2003.

[6]Ottesen G.L. Carcinoma in situ of the female breast. A clinico-pathological, immunological, and DNA ploidy study. APMIS Suppl. 108: p. 1-67, 2003.

[7]Lerner Barron H. Great expectations: historical perspectives on genetic breast cancer testing. Am. J. Pub. Health. 89: p. 938, 1999.

[8]James Vogel, M.D. personal communication.

[9]Fournier D., Weber E., Hoeffken W., Bauer M., Kubli F., and Barth V. Growth rate of 147 mammary carcinomas. Cancer 45: p. 2198, 1980.

[10]Fournier D. op. cit. p. 2205.

[11]Fournier D. op. cit. p. 2198.

[12]Horan A.H. Poster: Cancer of the prostate as an exponential function. See alpineurology.com.

[13]Ernester V.L., Barclay J, Kerlikowske K. et al Incidence of and treatment for ductal carcinoma in situ of the breast. JAMA 275: p. 913, 1996.

[14]Page D.L., Dupont W.D., Rogers L.W. et al. Continued local recurrence of carcinoma 15-25 years after diagnosis of low grade ductal carcinoma in situ of the breast treated only with biopsy. Cancer 76: p. 1197, 1995.

[15]Parens E. Glad and terrified: on the ethics of BRCA1 and BRCA2. Cancer Invest. 14: p. 405, 1996.

[16]Braun S., Pantel K., Muller P., Janni Wolfgang, Hepp F., Kentenich C., Gastroph S., Wischnik A., Dimpfl T., Kendermann G., Riethmuller G., and Schlimok G. Cytokeratin-positive cells in the bone marrow and survival of patients with stage 1,2, and 3 breast cancer. NEJ. 342: p. 525, 2002.

[17]Braun S., Pantel K., Muller P., Janni Wolfgang, Hepp F., Kentenich C., Gastroph S., Wischnik A., Dimpfl T., Kendermann G., Riethmuller G., and Schlimok G. Cytokeratin-positive cells in the bone marrow and survival of patients with stage 1,2, and 3 breast cancer. NEJ. 342: p. 525, 2002.

[18]Overgaard M., Hansen P.S., Overgaard J., at al Postoperative radiotherapy in high-risk premenopausal women with breast cancer who receive adjuvant chemotherapy. N. Eng. J. Med. 337: p. 956, 1997.

[19]Walsh P.C. Editorial comment on D.V. Fournier et al. Growth rate of 147 mammary carcinomas. Cancer 45: p. 2198, 1980. in J. Urol. 154: p. 1583, 1995.

[20]Lindeman F., Schlimok G., Dirschedl P., Witte J., Riethmuller G., Prognostic significance of micrometases in patients with gastric cancer. Lancet 340: p. 685, 1992.

[21]Jauch K.W., Heiss M.M., Gruetzner U. et al Prognostic significance of bone marrow micrometastases in patients with gastric cancer. J. Clin. Oncol. 14:p. 1810, 1996.

[22]Pantel K., Izbicki J.R., Passlick B., et al Frequency and prognostic significance of isolated tumor cells in bone marrow or patients with non-small-cell lung cancer without overt metastases. Lancet 347: p. 649, 1996.

[23]Machens A., Niccoli-Sire P., Hoegel J, *et al* Early malignant progression of hereditary medullary thyroid cancer. N.E.J. 349: p. 1517, 2003. Prophylactic thryroidectomy is being done but has not been proven to extend life.

[24]Martinez-Tello F.J., Martinez-Caruja R., Fernandez-Martin J., Losso-Oria C., Ballestin-Carcavilla C. Occult carcinoma of the thyroid. A systematic autopsy study from Spain of two series performed with two different methods. Cancer 71: p. 4022, 1993.

[25]Pelizzo M.R., Piotto A., Rubello D., Casara D., Fassina A., Busnardo B. High prevalence of occult papillary thyroid carcinoma in a surgical series for benign thyroid disease. Tumori 76: p. 255, 1990.

[26]Woods W.G., Ru-Nie G., Shuster J.J., Robison L.L., Bernstein M., Weitzman S., Bunin G., Levy I., Brossard J., Dougherty G., Tuchman M., Lemieux B. Screening of infants and mortality due to neuroblastoma. NEJ. 346: p. 1041, 2002.

[27]Schilling F. H., Spix C., Berthold F., Erttmann R., Fehse N., Hero B., Klein G., Sander J., Schwarz K. Treuner J., Zorn U., and Joerg M. Neuroblastoma screening at one year of age. NEJ 346: p. 1047, 2002.

[28]Kolata G. Screenings found harmless tumors while missing deadly cancers, studies say N.Y. Times 4/4/2002.

[29]Rockey D. C. Correspondance re virtual colonoscopy to screen for colon cancer. JEJM 350: p. 1148, 2004.

[30]Roehrborn C.G. The potential of serum prostate-specific antigen as a predictor of clinical response in patients with lower urinary tract symptoms and benign prostatic hyperplasia. BJU Int. suppl. 1: p. 21, 2004.

[31]Pavelic J., Zelk A. and Bosnar M.H. Molecular genetic aspects of prostate transition zone lesions. Urology 62: p. 607, 2003.

[32]The public calls this a 'rotorutor' job.

[33]Horan A.H. Learn to do the transurethral resection of the prostate with both hands…3 min. round Table, Western Section of the Am. Urol. Assoc. 11/93

[34]Hood H. M., Burgess P.A., Holtgrewe H. L., Fleming B., Mebust W., and Connolly R.P. Adherence for agency for health care policy research guidelines for benign prostatic hypertrophy. J. Urol. 158: p. 1417, 1997.

[35]Peterson's Urologic Pathology p. 608, 1992.

[36]Roehrborn C.G. PSA: A new role in the assessment and treatment of patients with LUTS and BPH. Reviews in Urology Supplement. 1999, p. 12.

[37]Pontes J.E. *et al* Serum prostatic antigen measurement in localized prostate cance: correlation with clinical course. J. Urol. 128: 1216, 1982.

[38]Roehrborn C.G. at al Serum prostate specific antigen is a strong predictor of future prostate growth in men with benign prostatic hyperplasia. J. Urol. 163: p. 13, 2000.

[39]Hochberg D.A., Basillotte B., Frachia J. A. Prostate specific antigen as a surrogate for prostate volume in patients with biopsy proven benign prostatic hyperplasia. J. Urol. 161, Supp.: p. 287, 1999.

[40]Basilotte J. B., Hochberg D.A., and Frachia J.A. A comparison of suprapubic versus transrectal ultrasonography in assessing prostatic volume in patients with biopsy proven benign prostatic hyperplasia (BPH) and prostate cancer (CaP). J. Urol. 161: No. 4. supplement, 1999.

[41]Horan A.H. BPH>150 grams in patients older than 75 years: is vaporization safe? Poster session Western Section A.U.A Kuai, Hawaii 10/25/02. Reported in Urology News.

[42]Horan A.H. Peak flow rates in the home with telephone reports. Does it build patient confidence in the indications for cystoscopy and prostatectomy? # min. North Central Section of the A.U.A. Orlando Fl. 11/18/88.

[43]Stamey et al. op. cit. NEJ 317, # 15, Oct 8, 1987, p. 909.

[44]Harris, G. "U.S. Panel Says No to Prostate Screening for Healthy Men" N.Y. Times   Oct. 6, 2011

[45]Kolata G. "A screening procedure for prostate cancer proves fallible." N.Y. Times Sunday, May 30, 2004. wk p. 7.

[46]Overmeyer M. "Men embrace PSA test but are they overly enthusiastic? Urology Times 32(4): p. 1, 2004.

[47]Chapman S. Fresh Row over prostate screening BMJ 326: p. 605, 2003.

[48]Yamey G. and Wilkes M. The PSA Storm. BMJ 324: p. 431, 2002

[49]Kolata Ibid

[50]Wang M.C., Valenzuela L.A., Murphy G.P., and Chu T.M. Purification of human prostate specific antigen.(Reprinted with permission from Invest. Urol. 17: p. 159, 1979.) in J. Urol. 167: p. 960, 2002

[51]Horan A.H. False positive PSA ascribed to B-cell lymphoma Poster. Western Section A.U.A. San Diego, 8/96.

[52]Hara M., Koyanazi T., Inoue T. et al Some physiochemical aspects of "gamma seminoprotein" and antigenic component specific for human seminal plasma. Jap. J. Legal Med. 25: p. 322, 1971.

[53]Stemey T.A. Preoperative serum prostate-specific antigen as a serum marker for adenocarcinom of the prostate. N. Eng. J. Med. 317: 909, 1987.

[54]Stamey op. cit. p. 915.

[55]Stamey T.A., Yang N., Hay A.R., et al Prostate specific antigen (PSA) below 10 microg/l predicts neither the presence of prostate cancer nor the rate of postoperative PSA failure. J. Clin. Chem. 47: p. 631, 2001.

[56]Stamey T.A. Personal communication, Oct. 25, 1999.

[57]Lange P.H. Editorial comment: J. Urol. 167: p. 965, 2002.

[58]Zlotta A.R. et al Prostate cancer and prostate specific antigen (PSA) levels: what is the PSA limit which reflects the prostate cancer itself and not the amount of benign tissue anymore? J. Urol. 169: supple. No. 4.p. 276, 2003.

[59]Sheikh K. and Bulllock C. Rise and fall of radical prostatectomy rates from 1989 to 1996. Urology 59: p. 379, 2002..

[60]Li J. op. cit. p 1786.

[61]Chang P. J. "Evaluating imaging test performance: an introduction to Bayesian analysis for urologists. Monographs in Urology. T. Stamey Editor . 12(2) Medical Directions Publishing Co. Inc. West Point, PA.p. 31. 1991.

[62]Punglia R.S. et al Effect of verification bias on screening for prostate cancer by measurement of prostate specific antigen. N.E.J. M. 349: p335, 2003.

[63]Schroder F.H. and Kranse R Verification bias and the prostate-specific antigen test—Is there a case for a lower threshold for biopsy? N.E.J.M. 349: p. 393, 2003. He cites the post-war paper of Franks L.M. Latent carcinoma of the prostate. J. Pathol. Bacteriol. 1954;68,603-16.

[64]Punglia et al point refer to a study by Morgan et al that achieved an area under the curve of .91 to .94. by selecting a population with a high prospective probability for cancer. op. cit. p. 340.

[65]Andriole G.L. Treatment with finasteride preserves usefulness of prostate-specific antigen in the detection of prostate cancer: resultsof a randomized, double-blind, placebo-controled clinical trial. Urology 52: p. 195-202, 1998.

[66]www.beckman.com/products/testdetail/access/freepsa.asp

[67] Brawer M.K., Cheli C.D., Horninger W., Babaian R., Fritsche H., Lepor H., Tnaja S., Childs S., Stamey T., Sokoll L., Chan D., Partin A., Bartsch G. Results of a multicenter prospective evaluation of complexed PSA. Oct. 23rd, 11:00 a.m. Western Section of the A.U.A, Kuai, Hawaii, 2002.

[68] Walsh P.C. Editorial comment in Urological Survey re Feneley M.R. *et al* "Today men with prostate cancer have larger prostates." Urology 56: p. 839, 2000.

[69] Horinaga M., Nakashima J., Ishibashi M., Oya M., Ohigashi T., Marumo K., and Murai M. Clinical value of prostate specific antigen base parameter for the detection of proste cance on repeat biopsy: the usefulness of complexed porstate specific antigen adjusted for transition zone volume. J. Urol. 168: p. 986, 2002.

[70] Horinaga M., Nakashima J., Ishibashi M., Oya M., Ohigashi T., Marumo K., and Murai M. Clinical value of prostate specific antigen base parameter for the detection of proste cance on repeat biopsy: the usefulness of complexed porstate specific antigen adjusted for transition zone volume. J. Urol. 168: p. 986, 2002.

[71] Isono T., Tanaka T., Kageyam S. and Yoshiki T. Structural diversity of cancer related and non-cancer related prostate specific antigen. Clinical Chemistry 48:p. 2187, 2002.

[72] Panneck J., Marks L.S., Pearson J.D., Rittenhouse H. G., Chan D.W., Shery E.D., Gormley G.J., Subong E.N., Kelly C.A., Stoner E., and Partin A.W. Influence of finasteride on free and total serum prostate specific antigen levels in men with benign prostatic hyperplasia. J. Urol. 159: p. 449, 1998.

[73] Bankhead C. "New Ventures may help make up for lost revenue." Urology Times.32: p.22, Dec. 2004. 74 Bankhead op. cit. p. 23.

[75] Starr D.S. Legal Issues in Medicine. "Skipped biopsy leads to a malpractice suit." Renal and Urology News. May 2004, p34.

[76] Otis Brawley, professor of medical oncology and epidemiology at the Winship Cancer Institute of Emory University quoted by G.Kolata in "Confronting cancer; prostate cancer; death rate shows small drop. But is it treatment or testing. N.Y. Times, April 9, 2002.

[77] L.K. Altman quoting E. David Crawford of the University of Colorado Health Science Center in Denver. "Report suggests prostate screening tests less frequently for some patients. N.Y. Times. May 21, 2002.

[78] Roberts R.O., Bergstrahl E.J., Peterson N. R., Bostwick D.G., Lieber M.M. and Jacobsen S.J. Positive and negative biopsies in the pre-prostae specific antigen and prostate specific antigen eras, 1980-1997.

[79] Hyman A. Letter in N.Y. Times. "In November, I will celebrate the fifth anniversary of my radical prostatectomy, a celebration for which I thank my wife, my surgeon, and my PSA test." Science Desk N.Y. Times April 13, 2002.

[80] Horan A.H. PSA blood tests and prostate cancer. W.S.J. p. A-27, 5/9/00.

[81] Associated Press. Prostate screening for men over 75 questioned. W.S.J. Dec. #rd, 2003.

[82] Wilkinso S. and Chodak G. Informed consent for prostate specific antigen screening. Urology 61: p.2-4, 2003.

[83] Gann P.H. Informed consent for prostate-specific antigen testing. Urology 61: p. 5, 2003.

[84] Etzioni R., Penson D.F., Legler J.M. *et al* Overdiagnosis due to prostate-specific antigen screening: lesson from US. Prostate cancer incidence trends. J. Natl. Cancer Inst. 94: p. 981-990, 2002.

[85] Talcott J. A. What should patients be told before agreeing to a blood test that could change their lives. Urology 61: p. 9, 20003.

[86] MCGregor M., Hanley J.A., Boivin J.F. *et al* Screening for prostate cancer: estimating the magnitude of overdtection. Can. Med. Assoc. J. 159: p. 1368, 1998.

[87] Brawley O. W. Informed consent for prostate specific antigen screening. Urology 61: p. 11, 2003.

[88]Zappa M., Ciatto S., Bonardi R., *et al* Overdiagnosis of prostate carcinoma by screening: an estimate based on the results of Florence Screening Pilot Study. Ann. Oncol. 9: p. 1297, 1998. 89

[89]H. Ballentine Carter Informed Consent for prostate-specific antigen screening. Urology 61: p. 13, 2003.

[90]Thompson I.A, Carter Informed Consent for prostate-specific antigen screening. Urology 61: p. 15, 2003.

[91]Schroder F.H., Wildhagen M.F., and the ERSPC Study Group: screening for prostate cancer: evidence and perspectives. BJU Int. 88: p. 811, 2001.

[92]Wolff A.M.D. and Schorling J.B. Preferences of elderly men for prostate specific antigen screening and the impact of informed consent. J. Gerontol. Med. Sci.

53A: M 195-M200, 1998.

[93]Chapman S."Fresh row over prostate screening." BMJ 2003; 326:605 (15 March).

[94]www.firthlawfirm.com/medmalcases.htm

[95]www.vaaglaw.com/cases

[96]Merenstein D. "A piece of my mind. Winners and Losers." JAMA 291: p. 15-16, 2004.

[97]Konety B. "Why we need to continue screening for prostate cancer in men older than 65 years. AUA News Sept. 2007, p. 12.

[98]Kolata Gina "10 million women who lack a cervix get Pap tests." N.Y. Times 6/23/04.

[99]H. Gilbert Welch, M.D., M.P.H. Should I be tested for cancer. University of California Press. Berkley and Los Angeles. 2004. passim.

[100]H. Gilbert Welch, M.D., M.P.H. Should I be tested for cancer? U. California Press. Berkley, CA, 2004.

[101]Atlantic Monthly Oct. 24, 2004, p. 116.

[102]Middleton A.W. 2002 Health policy survey results. Western Section A.U.A.,

1950 Old Tustin Ave., Santa Ana, CA. 92705.

[103]Prostate specific antigen (PSA): best practice policy.www.guidelines.gov.

[104]Halpern E.J., Frauscher F., Strup E., Nazarian L.N., O'kane P., Gomella L.G. Prostate: high-frequency Doppler U.S. imaging for cancer detection. Radiology 225: p. 71, 2002.

[105]Rahmi O, Littrup P.J., Pontes J.E., Bianco F.J. contemporary impact of transrectal ultrasound lesions for prostate cancer detection. J. Urol. 172: p. 512-

14, 2004.

[106]Lippman H.R., Ghiatas A.A., Sarosdy M.F. Systematic transrectal ultrasound guided biopsy after negative digitally directed prostate biopsy. J. Urol. 147: p. 827, 1992.

[107]Emiliozzi P., Corsetti A., Tassi B., Federico G., Martin M., and Pansadoro V. Best approach for prostate cancer detection: a prospectice study on transperineal versus transrectal six-core prostate biopsy. Urology 61: p. 961, 2003.

[108]Appelwhite J.C., Matlaga B.R., McCullough D.L. Results of the 5 region prostate biopsy method: the repeat biopsy population. J. Urol. 168: p. 500, 2002.

[109]Crawford E.D. *et al* Clinical staging of prostate cancer: a computer simulated study of transperineal biopsy. BJU Int. 96: p. 999, 2005.

[110]Appelwhite J.C., Matlaga B.R., McCullough D.L. Results of the 5 region prostate biopsy method: the repeat biopsy population. J. Urol. 168: p. 500, 2002.

[111]Cookson M.S. Update on transrectal ultrasound-guided needle biopsy of the prostate. Mol. Urol. 4: p. 93, 2000.

[112]Salmon L. *et al*, Cretil France. Does a 21 prostate needle biopsies protocol improve the prediction of PT3 status, positive surgical margins and tumor localization on radical prostatectomy specimens. J. Urol. 171(4) Supple, p. 229, 2004.

[113]Crawford E.D. oral communication, seminar on cryosurgery Denver, CO, March 24, 2004.

[114]Appelwhite J.C. op. cit. p. 501.

[115]Sperandeo G., Sperandeo M., Morcaldi M., Caturelli E., Dimitri L., Camagna A. Transrectal ultrasonography for the early diagnosis of adenocarcinoma of the prostate: a new maneuver designed to improve the differentiation of malignant and benign lesions. J. Urol. 169: p. 607, 2003.

[116]Emoliozzi P., Corsetti A, Tassi B, Martini G.F, and Pansadoro V, Best approach for prostate cancer detection: a prospective study on transperineal versus transrectal six-core prostate biopsy. Urology 61: p. 961.

[117]Vis A.N., Boerma M.O., Ciatto S., Hoedemaeker R.F., Schroder F.H. and van der Kwast T.H., Detection of prostate cancer: a comparative study of the diagnostic efficacy of sextant transrectal versus sextant transperineal biopsy. Urology 56: p. 617, 2000.

[118]Emiliozzi P., Corsetti A., Tassi B., Federico G., Martin M., and Pansadoro V. Best approach for prostate cancer detection: a prospectice study on transperineal versus transrectal six-core prostate biopsy. Urology 61: p. 961, 2003.

[119]Kojima M., Hayakawa T., Saito T., Mitsuya H., and Hayase Y. Transperineal 12-core biopsy method in the detection of prostate cancer. Int. J. Urol. 8: p. 301, 2001.

[120]Brullet E., Guevara M.C., Falco J., Puig J., Prera A., Prats J., and Del Rosario J. Endoscopy 32: p. 792, 2000.

[121]Petrowski R.A., Griewe G.L., Schenkman N.S. Delayed life-threatening hemorrhage after transrectal prostate needle biopsy. Prostate Cancer Prostatic Disease 6: p. 190, 2003.

[122]Otaibi M.F.A, Al-taweel W, Herba S. and Aprikian A.G. Disseminated intravascular coagulation following transrectal ultrasound guided prostate biopsy. J. Urol. 171: p. 346, 2004.

[123]Thompson P.M., Pryor J.P., Williams J.P., Eyers D.E., Dulake C., Scully M.F., and Kakkar V. The problem of infection after prostatic biopsy: the case for the transperineal approach. Br. J. Urol. 54: p. 736, 1982.

[124]Durkee C.T. Clostridia sepsis following transperineal needle biopsy of the prostate. J. Urol. 125: p. 752, 1981.

[125]Lindert K.A., Kabalin J.N. and Terris M.K. Bacteremia and bacteriuria after transrectal ultrasound guided prostate biopsy. J. Urol. 164: p. 76, 2000.

[126]Lujan G.M., Borda P A., Gonzalez F., Cajigal R., de Vicente G., and Sanchez B.A. Adverse effects fo transrectal prostatic biopsy. Analysis of 303 procedures. Actas Urol. Esp. 25: p. 25, 2001.

[127]Fong I.W., Struthers N., Honey R.J., Simbul M., Boiseau D.A. A randomized comparative study of prophylactic use of trimethaprim-sulfamehtoxazole versus netilmycin-metronidazole in transrectal biopsy. J. Urol. 146: p. 794, 1991.

[128]Ruebush T.K., McConville J.H., Calia F.M. A double-blind study of trimethoprim-sulfamethoxazole prophylaxis in patients having transrectal needle biopsy of the prostate. J. Urol. 122: p. 492, 1979.

[129]Thompson P.M., Talbot R.W., Packham D.A., Dulake C. Br. J. Surg. 67: p. 127, 1980.

[130]Sharpe J.R., Sadlowski R.W., Finney R.P., Branch W.T., Hanna J.E. Urinary tract infection after transrectal needle biopsy of the prostate. J. Urol. 127: p. 255, 1982.

[131]Babaian R.J., Lowry W.L., and Finan B.F. Intraluminal antibiotic regimen for patient undergoing transrectal needle biopsy of the prostate. Urology 20: p. 253, 1982.

[132]Gustafsson O., Norming U., Nyman C.R., Ohstrom M. Complications following combined transrectal aspiration and core biopsy of the prostate. Scand J. Urol. Nephrol. 24: p. 249, 1990.

[133]Kappor D.A., Klimberg I.W., Malek G.H., Wegenke J.D., Cox C.E., Patterson A.L., Graham E., Echols R.M., Whalen E., and Kowalsky S.F. Single-dose ciprofloxacin versus placebo for prophylaxis during transrectal prostate surgery. Urology 52;p. 522, 1998.

[134]Janoff D.M., Skarecky D.W., McLaren C.E., and Ahlering T.E. Prostate needle biopsy infection after four to six dose Ciprofloxacin. Can. J. Urol. 7: p. 1066, 2000.

[135]Griffith B.C., Morrey A.F., Ali-Khan M.M., Canby-Hagino E., Foley J.P., and Rozanski T.A. Single dose levofloxacin prophylaxis for prostate biopsy in patients at low risk. J. Urol. 168: p. 1021, 2002.

[136]Lindert K. A., Kabalin J.N., and Terris M.K. Bacteremia and bacteriuria after transrectal ultrasound guided prostate biopsy. J. Urol. 164: p. 76, 2000.

[137]Jeon S.S., Woo S.H., Hyun J.H., Choi H.Y., Chai S.E. Bisacodyl rectal prepartatin can decrease infectious complications of transrectal ultrasound- guided prostate biopsy. Urology 62: p. 461, 2003.

[138]Edson R.S., Van Scoy R.E., Leary F.J. Gram-negative bacteremia after transrectal needle biopsy of the prostate. Mayo Clin. Proc. 55: p. 489, 1980.

[139]Lai F.C., Kennedy W.A., Lindert K.A. and Terris M.K. Effect of circumcision on prostatic colonization and subsequent bacterial seeding following transrectal ultrasound-guided prostate biopsies. Tech. Urol. 7: p. 305, 2001.

[140]Norberg M., Holmberg L. Haggman M., Magnusson A. Determinants of complications after multiple transrectal core biopsies of the prostate. Eur. Radiol. 6: p. 457, 1996.

[141]Gilead J., Borer A., Mainon N., et al Failure of ciprofloxacin prophylaxis for ultrasound guided transrectal prostatic biopsy in the era of multiresistant enterobacteriaceae. J. Urol. 161: p. 222, 1999.

[142]Tal R., Livine P.M., Lask D., and Baniel J. Empirical management of urinary tract infections complicating transrectal ultrasound guided prostate biopsy. J. Urol. 169: p. 1762.

[143]Irani J., Roblot F., Becq G.B., and Dore B. Acute bacterial endocarditis secondary to transrectal ultrasound-guided prostatic biopsy. Scand. J. Urol. 36: p.

156, 2002.

[144]Eposti P.L., Elman A., Norlen H. Complications of transrectal aspiration biopsy of the prostate. Scand. J. Urol. Nephrol. 9: p. 208, 1975.

[145]Harris L.F., Jackson R.T., Breslin J.A., and Alford R.H. Anaerobic septicemia after transrectal prostatic biopsy. Arch. Intern. Med. 138: p. 393, 1978.

[146]Sandvik A., and Stefansen D. Eschericia coli meningitis following prostate biopsy. Tidsskr Nor Laegeforen 102: p. 499, 1982.

[147]Merino A.J., Roderiguez P.A., Baranda M., Luenga F., Aguirre E. E. coli bacteremia and non-Clostridial crepitant cellulits after transrectal prostatic biopsy in a diabetic patient. Rev. Clin. Esp. 169: p. 271, 1983.

[148]Spencer R.C., Courtney S.P., Nicol C.D. Polymicrobial septicaemia due to clostridium difficile and Bacteroides fragilis. Br. Med. J. 289; P. 531, 1984.

[149]Teichman J.M., Tsang T., McCarthy M.P. Osteitis pubis as a complication of transrectal needle biopsy of the prostate. J. Urol 148: p. 1260, 1992.

[150]Krause R.D., Dowd J.B., Larsen C.R., Cuttino J.T. and Scholz F.J. Acute pyelonephritis after transrectal ultrasonographically guided biopsy of the prostate: diagnosis by computed tomography. Comput. Med. Imanging Graph. 16: p. 297< 1992.

[151]Brewster S.F., Rooney N., Kabala J., Feneley R.C. Fatal anaerobic infection following transrectal biopsy of a rare prostatic tumor. Br. J. Urol.72: p. 977, 1993.

[152]Brasilis K.G., Stephens D.A. Adductor myonecrosis following prostate biopsy. Adductor myonecrosis following prostate biopsy. Aust. N.Z. J. Surg.67: p. 900, 1997.

[153]Borer A., Gilad J., Sikuler E., Riesenberg K., Schlaeffer F., and Buskila D. fatal Clostridium sordellii ischiorectal abscess with septicemia complicating ultrasound-guided transrectal biopsy. J. Infect. 38: p. 128, 1999.

[154]Gilad J., Borer A., Maimon N. et al. Failure of ciprofloxacin prophylaxis for ultrasound guided transrectal biopsy in the era of multresistant enterobacteriaceae. J. Urol. 161:p. 222, 1999.

[155]Hasegawa T., Shimomura T., Yamada H., Ito H., Kato N., Hasegawa N., Asano I., Kiyoto H., Ike-moto I., Onodera S., Oishi Y. Fatal septic shock caused by transrectal needle biopsy of the prostate: a case report. Kansenshogaku Zasshi 76:p. 893, 2002.

[156]Koefoed-Nielsen J., Mommsen S. Ugeskr Laeger 165: p. 51, 2002.

[157]Tal R. op. cit. p.1763.

[158]Esposti P.L. op. cit. 1975.

[159]Wasson J.H., Bubolz T.A., Yao G.L., Barry M.J. Prostate biopsies in men with limited life expectancy. Eff. Clin. Prac. 5: p. 137, 2002.

[160]Roberts R., Bergstralh E.J., Peterson N.R., Bostwick D.G., Lieber M.M., and Jacobsen S.J. Positive and negative biopsies in the pre-prostate specific antigen eras, 1980-1997.

[161]Roberts R. op. cit. passim.

[162]Spector W.G. The mediation of altered capillary permeability in acute inflammation, J. Path. Bact. LXXII(1956) p. 367.

[163]Young H. The early diagnosis and radical cure of carcinoma of the prostate.(Reprinted with permission from the Bull. Johns Hopkins University. Vol. XVI. No. 175, p. 315, October 1905) J. Urol. 168: p. 914, 2002.

[164]Mebust W.K., Holtgrewwe H.L., Cockett A., Peters P.C., and Writing committee. Transurethral prostatectomy: immediate and postoperative complications. Cooperative study of 13 participating institutions evaluating 3885 patients. J. Urol. 167: p. 5. 2002 (reprinted from 1989)

[165]Lerner B.H. Public Health Then and Now. Great Expectations: Historical Perspectives on Genetic Breast Cancer Testing. Am. J. Public Health 89: p. 938, 1999.

[166]Li C. Y., Shan S., Cao Y. and Dewhirst M.W. Role of incipient angiogenesis in cancer metastais. Cancer and Metastasis Reviews. 19: p. 7-11, 2000.

[167]Hanahan D., Folkman J. Patterns and emerging mechanisms of the angiogenic switch during tumorigenesis. Cell 86: p. 353, 1996.

[168]Folkman J. the roel of angiogenesis in tumor growth. Semin. Cancer Biol. 3: p. 65, 1992.

[169]J. Vogel, M.D. personal communication, autumn 2003.

[170]Paulson D.F. Editorial Comment. J. Urol. 167: p. 947, 2002.

[171]Mohammad Amin, M.D., personal communication.

[172]Young H. op. cit. p. 920.

[173]Gleason D.F., Mellinger G.T., and the Veterans Administration Cooperative Urological Research Group. J. Urol. 167: p. 953, 2002. Reprinted from J. Urol. 111: p. 58, 1974.

[174]Byar D. Corle D. and the Veterans Administration Cooperative Urological Research Group. VAC-URG randomized trial of radical prostatectomy for stage I and II prostate cancer. Urology 1981; Suppl. 17: p. 7.

[175]Madsen P.O., Graverson P.H., Gasser T.C., and Corle D. Scand. J. Urol. Nephrol. , Suppl. 110: p. 99, 1988.

[176]Rich A.R. On the frequency of occurrence of occult carcinoma of the prostate gland. J. Urol. 33: p. 216, 1934.

[177]O'Malley K.J., Pound C.R., Walsh P.C., Epstein J.I. and Partin A.W. Influence of biopsy perineural invasion on long-term biochemical disease-free survival after radical prostatectomy. Urology 59: p. 85, 2002.

[178]Ellis W. J., Pfitznmaier J., and Colli J., Arfman E.W., Lange P.H., and Vessella R.L. The detection and isolation of prostate cells from peripheral blood and bone marrow. Research Forum.#139 7: 46 a.m. 10/26/02. Western Section, A.U.A. Kuai, Hawaii.

[179]Funke I. and Schraut W. Metanalysis of studies on bone marrow micrometastases: an independent progonsitic impact remains to be substantiated. J. Clin. Oncol. 16: p. 557, 1998.

[180]Pantel, I. and Izbicki , J. Passlick, B., Angstwurm, M. Haussinger, K. Thetter, O. *et al* Frequency and prognostic significance of isolated tumor cells in bone marrow of patients with non-small cell lung cancer without overt metastases. Lancet 347: p. 649, 1996.

[181]Schlimok, G., Funke, I., Pantel, K., Strobel, F., Lindeman, F., Witte, J. : Micrometastatic tumour cells in bone marrow of patients with gastric cancer: methodological aspects of detection and prognostic significance. Euro. J. Cancer 27: p. 1461, 1991.

[182]Pantel , K. and Otte, M.: Disseminated tumor cells: diagnosis, prognostic relevance, and phenotyping. Recent Results in Cancer Research. 158; P. 14, 2001.

[183]Weckerman D., Muller P., Wawroschedk F, Harzman R., Reithuller G., and Schlimok G. Disseminated cytokeratin positive tumor cells in the bone marrow of patients with prostate cancer: detection and prognostic value. J. Urol. 166: p. 699, 2001.

[184]Mettlin C. Changes in patterns of prostate cancer care in the United States: results of American College of Surgeons Commission on cancer studies, 1974-1993.

[185]Sheikh K. and Bullock C. Rise and fall of radical prostatectomy rates from 1989 to 1996. Urology 59: p.378-382. 2001.

[186]Walsh P.C. and Donker P.J. Impotence following radical prostatectomy: insight into etiology and prevention. J. Urol. 167: p. 1005.

[187]Jencks S.F. and Wilensky G.R. The health care quality improvement initiative: a new approach to quality assurance in Medicare. J. Am. Med. Assoc. 268: p. 900, 1992.

[188]Sheikh K. and Bullock C. Effectiveness of interventions for reducing the frequency of radical prostatectomy procedures in the elderly. Am. J. Med. Qual. 18: p. 97, 2003.

[189]Bubolz T. op. cit. p. 978.

[190]Ellison L., Birkmeyer J. and Heaney J. National trends in the use of radical prostatectomy. J. Urol. 161: p. 36, 1999.

[191]It depends on the proper classification of cause of death of 6 patients. There were 6 fewer causes of "other deaths" in the watchful waiting group. But there is no reason that the watchful waiting group should have fewer "other deaths." If these 6 deaths are subtracted from the "cancer" caused deaths in the "watchful" group, the statistical significance is lost.

[192]Chirpaz E., Colonna M., Menegoz F., Grosclaude P., Schaffer P., Arveux P. , Leseac J.M., Exbrayat C. and Shearer R. Incidence and mortality trends for prostate cancer in 5 French areas from 1982 to 1996. Int. J. Cancer 97: p. 372, 2002.

[193]Medicare, non-HMO enrollees. Wennberg J. *et al*. The Dartmouth Atlas of Health Care. 1993. p. 55.

[194]Birmeyer J. D.*et al* Variation profiles of common surgical procedures. Surgery 124: p. 922, 1998.

[195]Skinner J, Weinstein J. N., Sporer S.M., and Wennberg J.E. Racial, ethnic, and geographic disparities in rates of knee arthroplasty among Medicare patients. N. Engl. J. Med. 349: p. 1350, 2003.

[196]Birkmeyer J. D., Sharp S.M., Finlayson S.R.G., Fisher E.S., and Wennberg J.E., Variation profiles of common surgical procedures. Surgery 124: p. 917, 1998.

[197]Brook R. H., Park R.E., Chassin M. R., Solomon D.H., Keesey J., and Kosecoff J. Predicting the appropriate use of carotid endarterectomy, upper gastrointestinal endoscopy, and coronary angiography. N.E.J. 323: p. 1173.

[198]Brook R.H. op. cit. p. 1176.

[199]Wennberg J. Which rate is right? N. Engl. J. Med. 314: p. 310, 1986.

[200]N.Y. Times, Sept. 17, 2000 As Electoral Vote Shapes Up..... p. 16.

[201] Lu-Yao G., McLerran D., Wasson J., Wennberg J. An assessment of radical prostatectomy. JAMA 269: p. 2633, 1993.

[202] Lu-Yao op. cit. p. 2635.

[203] Lai S. Lai, H., Krongrad A., Lam S., Schwade J., and Roos B. A. Radical prostatectomy: geographic and demographic variation. Urology 56: p. 114, 2000.

[204] G. Pezzino, Remington P.L., Anderson H. A., Harms L., Phillips J.L., Bruskewitz R. and Peterson D. Trends in surgical treatment of prostate cancer in Wisconsin, 1989-1991.

[205] Pezzino ibid.

[206] Shenghan L., Lai H., Lamm S., Obek C., Krongard A., and Roos B. Radiation therapy in non-surgically treated nonmetastic prostate cancer: geographic and demographic variation. Urology 57: p. 510, 2000.

[207] Wennberg op. cit. passim.

[208] Lai S. *et al* op. cit. passim.

[209] Lai S., Lai H., Krongrad A., Lamm S., Schwade J. and Roos B.A. Radical prostatectomy: geographic and demographic variation. Urology 56: p. 108, 2000.

[210] Lai S. *et al.* op. cit. p111.

[211] Method: data on the computer diskette supplied with the Dartmouth Atlas of Health Care was collated so that the hospital catchment areas in states comprising the Western Section of the A.U.A. could be compared to Northeast (defined as New England plus Pennsylvannia and New Jersey). Incomes, rates of teenage pregnancy, B.A. degrees, suicide, auto-accidents, and expenditures per capita for research and development by area were obtained from the Statistical Abstract of the United States, 1999. These were subjected to Peason correlations against radical prostatectomy. The estimate marginal means of measure were graphed and Pierson correlation coefficients calculated with BMDP Statistical Software (Cork Technology Park, Model Farm Rd. Cork Ireland, version 1990 (SUN/UNIX). In addition, pairwise comparison of mean rates of radical prostatectomy, breast sparing surgery, back surgery, and TURP in 1992 were also calculated with standard deviations and 'P' or 'r' values.

[212] Vitale M.G., Krant J.J., Gellins A., Heitjan D.F., Arons R., Bigliani L.U. and Flatow E. Geographic variation in the rates of operative procedures involving the shoulder, including total shoulder replacement, humeral head replacement, and rotator cuff repair. J. of Bone and Joint Surgery 81: p. 763, 1999.

[213] Lai S., Lai H., op. cit.

[214] Ernester V.L., Barclay J., Kerlikoski K., Grady D., Henderson C. Incidence of and treatment for ductal carcinoma in situ of the breast. JAMA 275: p. 913, 1996.

[215] Albain K. S., Green S.R., Lichter A.S., Hutchins L.F., Wood W.C., Henderson I.C., Ingle J. N., O'Sullivan J., Osborne C.K., Martino S. Influence of patient characteristics, socioeconomic factors, geography, and systemic risk on the use of breast-sparing treatment in women neroled in adjuvant breast cancer studies: an analysis of intergroup trials. J. Clin. Oncology 14: p. 3009. 1996.

[216] Lu-Yao G., Albertsen P.C., Stanford J. L., STukel T.A., Walkery-Corkery E.S., Barry M.J. Natural experiment examining impact of aggressive screening and treatment on prostate cancer mortality in two fixed cohorsts from Seattle area and Conn. BMJ 325: p. 740, 2002.

[217] Lai S., Lai H. , Krongrad A., Roos B.A. Overall and disease-specific survival after radical prostatectomy: geographic uniformity. Urology 57: p. 504, 2001.

[218] Angulo J. C., Akdas A., Eberle J. M., Haggman M., Malmstroom P., Pontes E.J., Sanchez-Chapado M., Turkert L., and Wodd D.P. Comparacion entre pacientes consideradatos para prostectomia radical en institutions academicas de distintos paises. Arch. Esp. de Urol 51: p. 959, 1998.

[219] Lynn Payer, Varieties of Treatment in the United States, England, West

Germany, and France. Henry Holt and Co. New York, 1996 forward p. xv.

[220]Fleshner N., Rakovitch E., and Klotz L. Differences between urologists in the Unitied States and Canada in the approach to prostate cancer. J. Urol. 163: p.1462.

[221]Fleshner N. op. cit. p. 1465.

[222]Chirpaz E., Colonna M., Menegoz F., Grosclaude P., Schaffer P., Arveux P., Lesech J. M., Exbrayat C., and Schaerer R. Incidence and mortality trends for prostate cancer in 5 French areas from 1982 to 1996. Int. J. Cancer 97: p. 372, 2002.

[223]Lynn Payer, Varieties of Treatment in the United States, England, West Germany, and France. Henry Holt and Co. New York, 1996. passim.

[224]Gilbert S.M. Wrongful Death. W.W. Norton New York: 1997. p.36-p.37.

[225]Lu-Yao R., McLerran D. , Wasson J. , Wennberg J.E. An assessment of radical prostatectomy. JAMA 269: p. 2633, 1993.

[226]Bubolz T., Wasson J.H., Lu-Yao G., and Barry M.J. Treatments for prostate cancer in older men: 1984-1997. Urology 58: p. 977, 2001.

[227]Factfinder.census.gov/servlet/QTTable?-ts=545.

[228]Karakiewicz P.I. et al Thirty day mortality rates and cumulative survival after radical retropubic prostatectomy. Urology 52(6): p. 1041-6, 1998.

[229]Sheikh K. and Bullock C. Rise and fall of radical prostatectomy rates from 1989 to 1996. Urology 59: p. 378, 2002.

[230]Hudson R. Brachytherapy treatments increasing among Medicare population.
Health Policy Brief. Sept. 1999. Am. Urol. Assoc. Baltimore, MD.

[231]Lu-Yao, op. cit.

[232]Horan A.H., Sohrabi K. and Mills P. The rise and fall of local therapy for prostate cancer in the San Joaquin Valley. Fed. Practitioner. April 1999.

[233]"PSA tests and prostate cancer." Letter in Wall Street Journal A-27, 5/9/00.

[234]Mushinski M. Prostate surgeries: average charges throughout the United States,
1997. Stat. Bull. Metrop. Insur. Co. 80: p. 10, 199.

[235]Fuer E.J., Merril R.M., and Hankey B.F. Cancer surveillance series: interpreting trends in prostate cancer—Part II: Case of death misclassification and the recent rise and fall in prostate cancer mortality. J. Nat. Cancer Inst. 91: p. 1030, 1999.

[236]Fuer op. cit.

[237]Stephenson R.A. and Merrill R.M. Prostate cancer trends from the SEER
database. A.U.A. News Sept. p. 23, 1999.

[238]Walsh P.C.Editorial comment on Tarone R.E. et al Implications of stage- specific survival rates in assessing recent declines in prostate cancer mortality rates. Empidemiology 11: p. 167-170, 2000.

[239]Meyer F., Moore L., Bairati I., Fradet Y., Downward trend in prostate cancer mortality in Quebec and Canada. J. Urol. 161: p. 1189, 1999.

[240]Albertson P. C., Walters S., and Hanley J.A. A comparison of cause of death determination in men previously diagnosed with prostate cancer who died in
1985 or 1995. J. Urol. 163: p. 519, 2000.

[241]Horan A.H. op. cit. BJU.

[242]Bubolz T. op. cit. 980.

[243]Fuer op. cit.

[244]Lu-Yao R. op. cit.

[245]Kiely T. "CDC holds international conference on prostate cancer."

[246]Cdc.gov/cancer/prostate

[247]"Changes in vitals etc. not reported: "window exit death" Busta v Columbus Hosp. Cor. 916P.2d 122-MMT (1996)

[248]B.M. Anonymous v. Drs. G. and P. *et al* County (MN) District Court, Case No. Kathleen Flynn Peterson at Robins, Kaplan, Miller, and Ciresi, Minneapolis, MN for plaintif. 06-96-8-3

[249]Valerie Wilkinson *et al* v. Ross Blades M.D. Smith-Glynn-Callaway Clinic. Green County (MO) Circuit Court Case No. 194CC2262. David W. Ansley of Ansley, Rodgers and Condry, Springfield MO for the plaintif.

[250]Demos M.P. Prostate specific antigen (PSA) and informed consent. AUA. News-May/June 1997, p. 30.

[251]Loretta Murray Vs. United States of America. 95-1523. Opinion to remand by Richard Posner. This was remanded for retrial on procedural issues. Politically, it was one of several operative misadventures that called into question the surgical services at North Chicago by the V.A. administrator at the time, former Congressman Derwinski.

[252]Kahan S.E., Goldman H. B., Marengo S., and Resnick M. Urological medical malpractice. J. Urol. 165: p. 1638, 2001.

[253]Available at website alpineurology.com.

[254]Stothers S. Vancouver B.C. 1996.

[255]Makinen T. *et al* Determining the cause of death in prostate cancer screening. J. Urol. 171(4) supple. p.472, 2004.

[256]Strasser H., Tienfenthaler M., Steinlechner M., t al: Urinary incontinence in the elderly and age-dependent apoptosis of rhabodosphincter cells. Lancet 354: p.918, 1999.

[257]Steer W.D. Modern management of urinary incontinence. AUA News June/July p. 18, 3003

[258]Mary Karr, "Sinners Welcome" in The Atlantic Monthly Oct. 4, 2004, p. 129.

[259]Kimberly Ford. Hump: True Tales of Sex after Kids. St. Martins Griffin. New York, 2008. passim.

[260]" The treatment he chose and I said I'd support was radiation and 'thought' we'd been told about the possible long term effects. Not So! Later I saw a vital, athletic, physical man feeling totally becoming afraid about, uninterested in our previous fabulous sex life...then depression. Deep. Sullen. Withdrawl from interests and from me...we grew farther and farther apart. My heart was breaking. I felt unattractive and rejected." A reader at Amazon.com

[261]Suh D.D. , Yang C.C., Cao Y. , Heeiman J., Garland P.A., Maravilla K.R. MRI of the Female Genital and Pelvic Organs during Sexual Arousal. Poster Session. Western Section A.U.A. Kuai, Hawaii, 2003, p. 40.

[262]Crouch N.S. *et al* Genital sensation after feminizing genitoplasty for congenital adrenal hyperplasia. BJU Int. 93: p. 135, 2004.

[263]Rupesh R. *et al* Long-term effect of sildenabil citrate on erectile dysfunction after radical prostatectomy: 3-year follow up. Urology 62(1): p. 110-115, 2003

[264]Raplh and Barbara Alterowitz. The Lovin' Ain't Over. Health Education Literary Publisher. Westbury N.Y. 1999, p.107.

[265]Savoie M., Kin S.S., Soloway M.S. A prospective study measuring penile length in men treated with radical prostatectomy for prostate cancer. J. Urol. 169: p. 1462, 2003

[266]Franken A.B. *et al*: what importance do women attribute to the size of the penis? Eur. Urol. 2002; 42: 426.

[267]Schober J.M. *et al* Self-Assessment of genital anatomy, sexual sensitivity, and function in women: implications for genitoplasty. BJU Int. 94: p. 589-594, 2004.

[268]Walsh P. C. Anatomical radical retropubic prostatectomy: detailed description of the surgical technique. J. Urol. 171: p. 2114, 2004.

[269]"Real Sex" on HBO Oct. 22, 2005.

[270]Eisenman R. Penis size: survey of female perceptions of sexual satisfaction. BMC Women's Health 1: p. 1, 2001.

[271]Rubiyat of Omar Kyam.

[272]Schulz W.W. , van Andel P., Sabelis I and Mooyart E. Magnetic resonance imaging of male and female genital during coitus and female sexual arousal. BMJ. 1999; 319: 1596.

[273]M. Korda's report on a men's group.

[274]Jackson G. Sexual intercourse and stable angina pectoris. Am. J. Cardiol. 86: p. 35-37, 2000.

[275]Raplh and Barbara Alterowitz. The Lovin' Ain't Over. Health Education Literary Publisher. Westbury N.Y. 1999, p.105.

[276]Angier, N. What do female bugs want? Surprise: it's shape, not size. N.Y. Times July 7, 1998.

[277]Angier N. New York Times article.

[278]Beutler L.E., Scott F. Brantley, Karacan I., Baer P.E., Rogers R.R., Morris J. Women's satisfaction with partners penile implant. Urology 24: p. 552, 1984.

[279]Montorsi F., Rigatti P., Carmingnani G., Giammusso B., Breda G., Mechanical reliability and patient-partner satisfaction with AMS three piece inflatable implants: a long-term multi-institutional study in 200 patients using Kaplan- Meier estimates. J. Urol. 159: p. 222, 1998.

[280]Usta M.F., et al Patient and partner satisfaction and long-term results after surgical treatment for Peyronie's disease. Urology 62: p. 105, 2003.

[281]Summer F. et al, Measurement of vaginal and minor labial oxygen tension for the evaluation of female sexual function. J. Urol. 165: p. 1181, 2001.

[282]Vardi Y., Gruenwald I. Sprecher E., Gertman I. and Yarnitsky D. Normative values for female genital sensation. Urology 56: p. 1035, 2000

[284]Blanchflower D.G. and Oswald A.J. Money, Sex and Happiness: an Empirical Study. Scandanavian Journal of Economics. July, 27, 2004, p. 9.

[285]Ibid. p. 10.

[286]Hilsenrath J.E. Pleasure principle: Study says more sex akin to higher pay.(quotes Blanchflower and Oswald above in second paper submitted to the National Bureau of Economic Research) Wall Street Journal Monday, June 7, 2004.

[287]Jane Juska A Round Healed Woman. Villard. New York. 2003.

[288]Jane Juska, A Round-Heeled Woman: My Late-Life Adventures in Sex and Romance. Villard

[289]Hisasue S., Kato R., Suzuki K., Shimizu T., Kobayashi K., Masumori N., Takahashi A., Itoh, N. Kamammoto Y, Tsukamota T. Impact of the partner's behavior on female quality of life: Japanese female chohort study. J. Urol. 169: supplement (4) p. 357, 2003.

[290]Smith J.S., Robertson C.N., Clipp E.C., Iden D., Lipkus I.M. Longitudinal assessment of quality of life and disease uncertainty in patients undergoing radical prostatectomy and spouses/partners. J. Urol. 169: Supple.(4) p. 34, 2003.

[291]John M. Barry, M.D., Ten things your urologist may not have told you about your radical prostatectomy. Abstracts 83rd meeting of the Western Section of the A.U.A.Scottsdaile at Gainey Ranch p. 89. Nov.1st 2007.

[292]Hu J.C., Gold K.F., Pashos C L., Mehta S.S., Litwin M.S. Temporal trends in radical prostatectomy complications from 1991 to 1998. J. Urol. 169: p. 1443, 2003.

[293]Kim Cattrell and Mark Levinson. Satisfaction. Warner Books. New York. 2002.

[294]Harlan L.C. et al Prostate cancer outcomes study: a population based study of the treatment of prostate cancer. J. Urol. 161: p. 37, 2000.

[295]Welsh J.S., Howard S.P., and Fowler J.F. Dose rate in external beam radiotherapy for prostate cancer: an overlooked confounding variable. Urology 62: p. 204, 2003

[296]Stobbe C.C. et al The radiation hypersensitivity of cells at mitosis. Int. J. Radiat. Oncol. Biol. Phys. 78: p. 1149, 2002.

[297]Wang J.Z. et al How low is the alpha/beta ratio for prostate cancer? Int. J. Radiat. Oncol. Biol. Phys. 55: p. 194, 2003.

[298]Zellweger T. et al Enhanced radiation sensitivity in prostate cancer by inhibition of the cell survival protein clusterin. Clin. Cancer Res.8: p. 276,2002.

[299]Zellweger et al Enhanced radiation sensitivity in prostate cancer by inhibition of the cell survival protein clusterin. Clin. Cancer Res. 8 (10) p. 3276, 2002.

[300]Sarosody M.F. Urinary and rectal complications of contemporary prostate brachytherapy (PB) for prostate cancer. J. Urol. 169: p.491, 2003

[301]Freiha F. External beam radiation therapy for cancer of the prostate. Mediguide to Urology 2(3) p. 8, 1987 Lawrence DellaCorte Publications, 919 Third Avenue, New York, N.Y. 10022.

[302]Wheeler J.A. et al Dedifferentiation of locally recurrent prostate cancer after radiation therapy. Presented at the 74th annual meeting of the American Radium Society, Orlando, Florida, April 11-15th, 1992 for the M.D. Anderson Center Dept of Radiotherapy.

[303]Stamey T.A. et al The value of serial prostate specific antigen determinations 5 years after radiotherapy: steeply increasing value characterize 80% of patients. J. Urol. 150: p. 1856, 1993.

[304]Kuettel M. et al Radiation induced malignant transformation of a human prostate epithelial cell line. (267B1) J. Urol. 155: p. 607A, 1996.

[305]Grossfeld G.D. et al Locally recurrent prostate tumors following either radiation therapy or radical prostatectomy have changes in KI-67 labelling index, P53 and BCL-2 immunoreactivity. J. Urol. 159: p. 1437, 1998.

[306]Winters J.C. and Fuselier H.A. Invasive bladder cancer following I 125 implants. J. Urol. 148: p. 1898.

[307]Yurdakul G. et al Rectal squamous cell cancer 11 years after brachytherapy for carcinoma of the prostate. J. Urol. 169: 280, 2002.

[308]Navon J.D. et al. Angiosarcoma of the bladder after therapeutic irradiation for prostate cancer. J. Urol. : p. 1359, 1997.

[309]Sarosody M. op. cit. 2003.

[310]Pesce et al Vesico-crural and vesicorectal fistulas 13 years after radiotherapy for prostate cancer. J. Urol. 168: p. 2118, 2002.

[311]Robinson J.W. et al Meta-analysis of erectile function after treatment of localized prostate carcinoma. Int. J. Radiat. Oncol. Biol. Phys. 54: p. 1063, 2002.

[312]Atlantic Monthly, July-August 2003, p.35.

[313]Sarosody M. Pulmonary seed migration after permanent transperineal prostate brachytherapy is relatively common. J. Urol. (4) Supple p. 282, 2004.

[314]Grove A. Fortune, May 13, 1996, p. 55.

[315]Christine Jacobs, Key presentations report best ever results in 5-10 year cure rates: fewer, less severe side effects compared to other therapies. Business Wire, Buford GA, Oct. 17, 2002.

[316]Gray C. et al 20- year outcome of patients with T1-3N0 surgically staged prostate cancer treated with external beam radiation therapy. J. Urol. 166: p. 116, 2001.

[317]Cornelius Ryan and Cathryn Morgan Ryan. A Private Battle. Simon and Schuster. New York: 1979, p. 184.

[318]Stamey T.A. Letter in reply to a letter by I. Kaplan and C. Coleman re "The value of serial prostate specific antigen determinations 5 years after radiotherapy: steeply increasing value characterize 80% of patients. J. Urol. 152: p. 494, 1994.

[319]Neoptolemos J.P. *et al.* A randomized trial of chemradiotherapy and chemotherapy after resection of pancreatic cancer. N.E.J.M. 350: p. 1200, 2004. The editorialist in the same issue M. Choti stuggled to say that radiation made the cancer worse but says it eventually.

[320]Corporate-ir.net/ireye/ir

[321]Theragenics TM Annual report, p. 5.

[322]Eccles S.A. and Welch D.A. Metastasis: recent discoveries and novel treatment strategies. The Lancet 369: p. 1742, May 19, 2007. 1a Morgan T.M. *et al* Disseminated tumor cells in prostate cancer: implications for systemic progression and tumor dormancy. J. Urol. 177: No 4: p. 220, 2007.

[323]Olson C.A. Circulating prostate derived cells in patients with prostate adenocarcinoma. J. Urol. 163: p. 1631, 2000.

[324]Ng J.C., Koch M.O., Daggy J. K., and Cheng L. perineural invasion in radical prostatectomy specimens: lace of prognostic significance. J. Urol. 172: p. 2249, 2004.

[325]Debbage P., Strohmeyer D., Wieser E., Rogatasch H. Horninger W., Bartsch G. How does PSA leak into the blood? Fine structural changes of microvasculature in prostate cancer. Abst. J. Urol. 169 (4) Suppl. P. 154, 2003.

[326]Huang W., Chung L.W. Invasive prostate cancer cells secrete soluble protein fctors that upregulate osteocalcin(OC) promoter activity: implication to stroma desmoplastic response and cancer metastasis. J. Urol. 169 (4) Suppl. P. 154, 2003.

[327]Ahmann F.R., Woo L., Hendrix M., Trent J.M. Growth in semisolid agar of prostate cancer cells obtained from bone marrow aspirates. Cancer Research 46: p. 3560, 1986.

[328]Mansi J.L., Berger U., Wilson P., Shearer R., Coombes R.C. Detection of tumor cells in the bone marrow of patients with prostatic carcinoma by immunocytochemical means. J. Urol. 139: p. 545, 1988.

[329]Riesenberg R., Oberneder R., Kriegmair M., Epp M., Bitzer U., Hofstetter A., Braun S., Riethmuller G., Pantel K. Immunocytochemical double staining of cytokeratin and prostate specific antigen in individual prostatic tumor cells. Histochemistry 99: p. 61, 1993.

[330]Bretton P.R., Melamed M.R., Fair W.R. Cote R.J. Detection of occult micrometastases in the bone marrow of patients with prostate carcinoma. Prostate 25: p. 108, 1994.

[331]Oberneder R., Riesenberg R., Kriegmair M., Bitzer U., Klammert R., Schneede P., Hofstetter A., Riethmuller R., and Pantel K. Immunocytochemical detection and phenotypic characterization of micrometastatic tumor cells in the bone marrow of patients with prostate cancer. Urological Research. 22: p. 3, 1994.

[332]Pantel K., Schlimok G., Angstwurm M., Weckermann D., Schmaus W., Gath H., Passlick B., Izbicki J.R., Riethmuller G. Methodological analysis of immunocytochemical screening for disseminated epithelial tumor cells in the bone marrow. J. of Hematotherapy 3: p. 165, 1994.

[333]Coli J. L., Ellis W.J., Arfman E.W., Lange P. H., Vessella R.L. The detection and isolation of prostate cancer cells from peripheral blood and bone marrow. Abst. A.U.A. Anaheim CA, June, 2000.

[334]Ellis W.J., Pfitzenmaier J, Janet Colli, Arfman E., Lange P.H. and Vessela R.L. Detection and isolation of prostate cancer cells from the peripheral blood and bone marrow. Urology 61: p. 277, 2003.

[335]Lin D. *et al* Detection and isolation of PSA positive epithelial cells by enrichment: comparison to standard PSA RT-PCR, clinical relevance and initial characterization in prostate cancer patients. J. Urol. 171: p. 221, 2004.

[336]Forelle C. Test predicts breast cancer survival. WSJ, Thursday, 8/19/04.

[337]Miller M.C. *et al* Circulating tumor cells (CTCs) predict survival in patients with metastatic prostate cancer. Poster session. American Association for Clinical Research, Orlando, FL, March 2004.

[338]Okegawa T. *et al* Immunomagnetic Quantification of Circulating Tumor Cells as a Prognostic Factor of Androgen Deprivation Responsiveness in Patient with Hormone Naïve Metastatic Prostate Cancer. J. Urol. 180: p. 1342, 2008.

[339]E.C. Kauffman, V.L. Robinson, W.M. Stadler, M.H. Sokoloff and C.W. Rinker- Schaeffer "Metastases suppression: evolving role of metastasis suppressor genes for regulating cancer cell growth at secondary site. Investigative Urology in J. Urol. 169: p. 1124, 2003.

[340]Katz A.E., Olisson C.A., Raffo A., Cama C., Perlman H., Seaman E., O'Toole K., McMahon D., Benson M.C. and Buttan R. Molecular staging of prostate cancer with the use of an enhanced reverse transcriptase-PCR assay. Urology 43: p. 765, 1994.

[341]Polascik T.J., Wang Z., Shue M., Di S., Gurganus R.T., Hortopan S.C., Ts'O P., and Partin A. W. Influence of sextant prostate needle biopsy or surgery on the detection and harvest of intact circulating prostate cancer cells. J. Urol. 162: p. 749, 1999.

[342]Katz A.E., de Vries G.M., Beg M.D., Raffo A., Cama C., O'toole K., Buttyan R.E., Benson M.C., and Olsson C.A. Enhanced reverse transcriptase- polymerase chain reaction for prostate specific antigen as an indicator of true pathologic stage in patients with prostate cancer. Cancer 75: p. 1642, 1995.

[343]Edelstein R.A., Zietman A.L., de las Morenas A., Krane R.J., Babayan R.K., Dallow K.C. *et al* Implications of prostate micrometastases in pelvic lymph nodes: an archival tissue study. Urology 47: p. 370, 1996.

[344]Weckerman D., Muller P., Wawroschek F., Harzmann T., Riethmuller G., and Schlimok G. Disseminated cytokeratin positive tumor cells in the bone marrow of patients with prostate cancer detection and prognostic value. J. Urol. 166: P. 699, 2001.

[345]Gewanter R.M., Katz A.E., Olsson C.A., Benson M.C., Singh A., Schiff P.B. and Ennis R.D. RT-PCR for PSA as a prognostic factor for patients with clinically localized prostate cancer treated with radiotherapy. Urology 61: p. 967, 2003.

[346]Gao C.L., Rawal S.K., Sun L. Ali A., Connelly R., Banez L., Sesterhenn I.A., McLeod D.G. Moul J. W. and Srivastava S. Diagnostic portential or prostate specific antigen expressing epithelial cells in the blood of prostate cancer patients. Clin. Cancer Res. 7: p. 2545, 2003.

[347]Katz A. personal communication Duke Urological Symposium. Feb. 28, 2004

Park City Utah. 348 Harisinghani M.G. *et al* Noninvasive detection of clinically occult lymph-node metastases in prostate cancer. N.E.J. M.

[348]p. 2491, 2003.

[349]Rogers J. The course of acquired disease of the thyroid gland and the principles which seem to control its progress. Annals of Surgery. P. 281, 1914.

[350]Rutherforod R, Erisman E., Daly S., Practice management tips 3: American Urological Association, 1000 Linthicum M.D. 21090, 2004. p. 16.

[351]Personal communication via e-mail. HommoYukia, 11/14/04.

[352]Matsuo H., Baba Y., Nair R.M.G., Arimura A., and Schally A.V. Structure of the porcine LH- and FSH-releasing hormone. 1. The proposed amino acid sequence. (Reprinted with permission from Biochem. Biophys. Res. Comm, 43: p.1334, 1991.

[353]Nicholas Wade, The Nobel Duel, Anchor Press/Doubleday, Garden City, N.Y., 1981.

[354]Guillemin R. Hypothalamic hormones a.ka. hypothalamic releasing factors. J. Endocrinology 184: p. 11, 2005.

[355]Keyes E.L. and Ferguson R.S.. Urology, 6th ed. New York: D. Appleton- Century, pp. 425-426, 1936.

[356]Counseller V.S. Proceeding of Mayo Clinic Staff meeting. Proc. Mayo Clin. 11: p. 788, 1936.

[357]Lytton B. Prostate cancer: a brief history and the discovery of hormonal ablation treatment. J. Urol. 165: p. 1859, 2001.

[358]Huggins C. and Hodges C. The effect of castration, of estrogen, and of androgen injection on the serum phosphatases in metastatic carcinoma of the prostate. Reprinted with permission from Cancer Res. 1: p. 293, 1941, in J. Urol. 167: p. 948, 2002.

[359]Byar D.P. Studies of carcinoma of the prostate. The Veterans Administration Cooperative Urological Research Group studies. Cancer 32: p. 1162, 1973.

[360]tap.com/about/financials

[361]Isaacs J. T. The timing of androgen ablation therapy and/or chemotherapy in the treatment of prostatic cancer. The Prostate 5: p. 1-17, 1984.

[362]Isaacs J. T. The timing of androgen ablation therapy and/or chemotherapy in the treatment of prostatic cancer. The Prostate 5: p. 1-17, 1984.

[363]Medical Research Council Prostate Cancer Working Party. Immediate versus deferred treatment for advanced prostate cancer: initial results of the the Medical Research Council Trial. Br. J. Urol. 79: p. 235, 1997.

[364]Messing E., Manola J., Sarosdy M., Wilding G., Crawford E.D., and Trump D.

Immediate hormonal therapy compared with observation after radical prostatectomy and pelvic lymphadenectomy in men with node positive prostate cancer. N.E.J. 341: p. 1781, 1999.

[365]Wirth M. *et al* Bicalutamide (Casodex) 150 mg as immediate therapy in patients with localized or locally advanced prostate cancer significantly reduces the risk of disease progression. Urol. 58: p. 146, 2001.

[366]Holzbeierlein J., Payne R., Weigel J., and Mardis H. Long-term followup of metastatic prostate cancer. J. Urol. 171: p. 2377, 2004.

[367]Akaza H. Efficacy of hormone therapy for localized and locally advanced prostate cancer: results of 10-year follow up. J. Urol. 175: p. 212, 2006.

[368]Homma Yukio. E-mail, Nov. 9th, 2004, 1:35 a.m.

[369]Astra-Zeneca website.

[370]Horan A. H. Fractures ascribable to osteoporosis following LHRF antagonism for carcinoma of the prostate; a preliminary survey. Poster. Western Section A.U.A. Seattle WA 8/25/94.

[371]Bankhead C. quoting M. Garnick M.D. at the American Society of Clinical Oncology Meeting. "Androgen deprivation therapies prolong QT interval. Urology Times. Sept. 2004. p. 22.

[372]Mac Overmyer, Short term androgen therapy plus RT boost survival. Urology

Times. 32, No 14, Oct. 2004, p. 1.

[373]Encyclopedia Brittanica Chicago, 1954, Volume 4, p. 555.

[374]Coffey D.S. and Isaacs J.T. "Experimental concepts in the design of new treatments for human prostate cancer. Chapter XIV in Prostate Cancer: A series of workships on the biology of human cancer. Int. Union against Cancer. Geneva

1979. p. 233.

[375]Charbit A., Malaise E.P., and Tubiana M. Relation between the pathological nature and growth rate of human tumors. Europ. J. Cancer 7: p. 307, 1971. 376

[377]Horan, A.H. Brit. J. Urol. op. cit.

[378]Fidler I.J. "Molecular biology of cancer: invasion and metastasis" in Principle and Practice of Oncology, Lippincott-Raven, Philadelphia, p. 141, 1997.3

[379]Noldus J. and Stamey T.A. J. Urol. 155, p 441, 1996.

380 www.bankrate.com/calculator.`````````````````````````````

[381]Zwergel U. *et al* Lymph node positive prostate cancer: long-term survival data after radical prostatectomy. J. Urol. 171: p. 1128, 2004.

[382]Khan M.A., Partin A.W., and Carter H. B. Expectant management of localized prostate cancer. Urology 62 p. 796, 2003.

[383]Isaacs J.T. response to

[384]Sacks O. Forward in Anatole Broyard, Intoxicated by my illness. Fawcett Columbine. 1992, p. xv,

[385]I know for example of a philosophy major who became a successful private practice urologist.

[386]Alexandra Broyard. Prologue. In Anatole Broyard, Intoxicated by my illness. Fawcett Columbine. 1992, p. xviii,.

[387]He overtly refers to French deconstruction later. "If I were to demystify or deconstruct my cancer, I might find that there is no absolute diagnosis, no single agreed-upon text, but only the interpretation each doctor and each patient makes." This book contests this point of view. There is an agreed upon text. This is it. The dispute rests upon the question of who must agree with it.

[388]Op cit p. 37.

[389]op. cit. p. 5.

[390]Op cit p. 121.

[391]Katheryn Morgan Ryan, "About Cornelius" in A Private Battle. Simon and Schuster, New York, 1979, p. 392 30 of the 90 patients used to justify the label for that drug came from my private practice. I 'published' a poster with Pfizer about this use and showed it at the American Geriatric Society.

392 Katheryn Morgan Ryan, "A Private Battle," Simon and Schuster, New York, 1979.

[393]Op. cit. p. 79.

394 Katheryn Morgan Ryan, "A Private Battle," Simon and Schuster, New York, 1979.

[395]Op cit. p. 86.

[396]Op.cit. p. 88.

[397]Isaacs J. Response to Horan A.H. "We should tell the patients the age of their cancers." A.U.A. News. July 2000. p. 23.

[398]Op cit. p. 161.

[399]Charbit A., Malaise E.P., and Tubiana M. Relation between the pathological nature and growth rate of human tumors. Europ. J. Cancer 7: p. 307, 1971.

[400]Stamey T.A. Letter. Radiotherapy "…may make the 80% that failed therapy worse…I hope that most physicians will recognize that radiotherapy is no longer a viable option for the treatment of prostate cancer." J. Urol. 152: p. 494, 1994.

[401]Katherine Ryan op. cit. p. 193.

[402]This is the work of the early Scottish philosopher David Hume. For Hume would say you cannot infer from animal studies, or even earlier studies in man because the nature of the universe may turn upside down while you are sleeping. You must do the experiment he said. This sounded rigorous in the early nineteenth century but it is nonsense to day. We acknowledge that at the subatomic level what happens is statistical, a role of the dice. Most of us acknowledge that as the muons and quarks aggregate in to larger clumps, their behavior become predictable with certainty. You would never know it from these accounts.

[403]Op. cit. p. 194.

[404]Katherine Morgan Ryan. Op. cit. p. 226.

[405]Nesbit R.M. Endocrine control of prostatic carcinoma. JAMA 143: p. 1317-1320, 1950.

[406]Veterans Administration Co-operative Urological Research Group: Treatment and survival of patients with cancer of the prostate. Surg. Gynecol. Obstet. 124: p. 1011, 1967.

[407]N.Y. Times 12/17/02

[408]Rasmussen L.S., Sperling B., Abildstrom H.H., Moller J.T. Neuron loss after coronary artery bypass detected by SPECT estimation of benzodiazepine receptors.

[409]Hall R.A., Fordyce D.J., Lee M.E., Eisenberg B., Lee R.F., Holmes J.H., and Campbell W.G. Brain SPECT imaging and neuropsychological testing in coronary artery bypass patients: single photon emission computed tomography. Ann. Thorac. Surg. 68: p. 2082, 1999.

[410] Johnson T., Monk T., Rasmussen L.S., Abildstrom H., Houx P., Korttila K., Kuipers H.M., Hanning C.D., Siersma V.D., Kristensen D., Canet J., Ibanaz M.T., Moller J.T., ISPOCD2 Investigators. Anesthesiology 96:p. 1351, 2002.

[411] Shelski F.D., Henley J.D., Foster R.S., and Einhorn L.H. Prostate carcinoma presenting as multiple pulmonary nodules in an asymptomatic patient with a history of testicular non-seminomatous germ cell tumor. Urology 62: p. 748, 2003.

[412] Horan, T. Bram "Causality, Necessity, and the Hum(e)an Mind." For Prof. Gabbey, April 17th, 2003.

[413] Horan, T.B. op. cit.

[414] "Controlled" means that there is an untreated group as well as a treated group. "Prospective" means that the rules of the experiment are pre-set and unchangeable during the experiment. "Randomized" means that who enters the experimental group and who enters the control group is set by chance, not the investigators.

[415] Bloom B.S. Controlled studies in measuring the efficacy of medical care: a historical perspective. The Journal of Technology Asssessment. P. 299. 198?

[416] Madsen P. O., Graverson P.H., Gasser T. C., and Corle D. Treatment of localized prostatic cancer. Radical prostatectomy versus placebo. A 15 year follow up. Scand. J. Urol. Nephrol., suppl. 110: P. 110, 1988.

[417] Iverson P., Madsen P.O., and Corle D. Radical prostatectomy versus expectant treatment for early carcinoma of the prostate. Twenty-three year follow up of a prospective randomized study. Scand. J. Urol. Suppl. 172: p. 65.

[418] Middleton R., Thompson I.A., Austenfeld M.S., Cooner W.H., Correa R.J., Gibbons R.P., Miller H.C., Oesterling J. E., Resnick M.I., Smalley S.R., Wasson J.H. Report on the management of clinically localized prostate cancer. A.U.A. July, 1995. p. i.

[419] Middleton R. op. cit. p. 42.

[420] Isaaacs_

[421] Middleton R. op. cit. p. 44.

[422] Middleton R. op. cit. p.35

[423] Middleton R. op. cit. p. 22.

[424] Franks L.M. Latent carcinoma of the prostate. J. Path. Bact. 68:p. 603, 1954.

[425] Sakr W.A., Haas G.P., Cassin B.F., Pontes J.E., Crissman J.D. The frequency of carcinoma and intraepithelial neoplasia of the prostate in oung male patients. J. Urol. 150: p. 379, 1993.

[426] Middleton R. et al op. cit. p. 19.

[427] Eddy D.M. A manual for assessing health practices and designing practice policies: the explicit approach. Philadelphia: Am. Coll. Of Physicians. 1992. p. 126.

[428] Middleton R. et al op. cit. p. 8.

[429] A=b, b=c, therefore a=c. Euclid's portability of equivalence.

[430] Resnick M.I. personal communication. 7/20/1998.

[431] OTA-BP-H-145, Washington, D.C. U.S. Government Printing Office, May 1995.

[432] OTA op. p. 4.

[433] OTA op. cit. p. 4

[434] OTA, op. cit. p. 8.

[435] Holmberg L. et al A randomized trial comparing radical prostatectomy with watchful waiting in early prostate cancer. NEJ 347: p. 781.

[436] Sample size for estimation of prevalence in a population. Stat page. Net- interactive stats. Dept. of Ob. Hong Kong.

437 Horan A.H., Nasrabadi K.S., and Mill P. Localized therapy for prostate cancer: private-versus public sector practice. Fed. Pract. April 1999.

438 Wilt T.J. *et al.* An evaluation of radical prostatectomy at Veteran Affairs medical centers. Med. Care 37: p. 1046, 1999.

439 Antidepressants and pediatric depression. N. Eng. J. Med. 351(16): p. 1599, 2004.

440 p. 202-203. Steven Pinker, The Blank Slate. Viking, New York: 2002.

441 An expression among political journalist to characterize a colleague who has become a friend of a candidate and therefore lost his objectivity.

442 McDade T. Prostates and Profits: the Social Construction of Benign Prostatic

Hyperplasia in American Men. Medical Anthropology 17: p. 1, 1996.

443 Fukuyama F. The Great Disruption. The Atlantic Monthly, May 1999, p. 55.

444 E-mail Sunday, April 11, 2004, 5:16 pm from Mohammad Amin.

445 You can spot a louse on someone else but you can't see the tick on yourself. A Natural History of Latin. Op.cit. p.282.

446 Studer-Ellis E, Gold J.S, Jones R.F. Trends in U.S. medical school faculty salaries, 1988-1989 to 1998-1999.

447 Jonas H.S., Etzel S.I., Barzansky B. Educational programs in U.S. medical schools. JAMA 270: p. 1061, 1993.

448 Blumenthal D. New steam from an old cauldron-the physician supply debate. N.E.J.M. 350: p. 1781, 2004.

449 Blumenthal op.cit. p. 1782, Table 1.

450 Abelson R. "Barred as rival, doctors see some hospitals in court. N.Y. Times.

4/13/04

451 Brook R.H., Park R.E., Chassin M.R., Solomon D.H., Keesey J., Kosecoff. Predicting the appropriate use of carotid endarterectomy, upper gastrointestinal endoscopy, and coronary angiography. NEJ 323: p. 1173, 1990.

452 Weindling P. The origins of informed consent: the international scientific commission on medical war crimes, and the Nuremburg code. Bull. Hist. Med.

75: p. 37, 2001.

453 The Nuremburg Code(from Trials of War Criminals before the Nuremburg Military Tribunals under Control Council Law N0. 10 Nuremburg, Oct. 1946- April 1949. Washington D.C. U.S.G.P.O. 1949-1953.#3.

454 "Authocthonous" means grown from the animal not implanted from another animal.

455 Henry J. M. and Isaacs J.T. Relationship between tumor size and the curability of metastatic prostatic cancer by surgery alone on in combination with adjuvant chemotherapy. J. Urol. 139: p. 119, 1988.

456 Plonowski A, Schally A.V., Nagy A., Sun B. Halmos G. Effective treatment of experimental DU-145 prostate cancers with targeted cytotoxic somatostatin analog AN-238. Int. J. Onco. 20: p. 397, 2002

457 Sonderegger-Iseli K., Burger S., Muntwyler J., Salomon F., Diagnostic errors in three medical areas: a necropsy study. Lancet 355:p. 2027, 2000.

458 Vidic B. and Weitlauf H.M. Horizontal and vertical integration of academic disciplines in the medical school curriculum. Clin. Anat. 15:p. 233, 2002.

459 Gillenwater J.Y. and Gray M. Evidence: what is it, where do we find it, and how do we use it? European Urology Supplements 2: p. 3, 2003.

460 Chodak G.W., Thistead R.A., Gerber G.S., Johansson J., Adolfsson J., Jones G.W., Chisholm G.D., Moskovitz, Livne P., and Warner J. Results of conservative management of clinically localized prostate cancer. N.E.J. 330: p. 242, 1994.

[461]7 medical schools were founded in the 1970s based on the Veterans Administration Hospitals.

[462]Kahn M.A., Partin A.W., and Carter H. Expectant management of localized prostate cancer. Urology 62: p. 796, 2003.

[463]Kenneth M. Ludmerer. Time to heal: American Medical Education from the turn of the century to the era of managed care. Oxford University Press. 1999. passim.

[464]Sheikh K. and Bullock C. Rise and fall of radical prostatectomy rates from 1989 to 1996. Urology 59(3) p. 378, 2002.

[465]Flemming C, Wasson J.H., Albertsen P.C., et al for the Prostate Patient Outcomes Research Team: A decision analysis of alternative treatment strategies for clinically localized prostate cancer. JAMA 269: p. 2650, 1993.

[466]Bubolz T., Wasson J.H., Lu-Yao G., Barry M.J. Treatment for prostate cancer in older men: 1984-1997. Urology 58: p. 977, 2001.

[467]McNett C.L." Legislative wrap up 2003: a year in review" Health Policy Brief 14 (1): p.3.

[468]Chase, Randal. Fresno Bee. "Drug maker to pay $355 m to settle case." June, 2003.

[469]McKay and Armstrong D. Advanced magnetics' stock surge spark investigation by AMEX. W.S.J. 6/19/2003.

[470]Ridge J. Law suits and mergers in managed care. Health Policy Brief Dec. 2003 Am. Urol. Assoc. Inc. 1000 Corporate Blvd., Linthicum, MD, 2109.

[471]Horan A.H.Sequential cryotherapy for carcinoma of the prostate: does it palliate the bone pain? Conn. Med. 39: p.81, 1975.

[472]Tunis S.R. Why Medicare has not established criteria for coverage decisions.

N.E.J. M. 350;(21) p. 2197, 2004.

[473]Dearnaley D.P., Kirby R.S., Kirk D., Malone P., Simpson R.J., and William G. Diagnosis and management of early prostate cancer: Report of a British Association of Urological Surgeons Working Party. BJU 83: p. 18, 1999.

[474]Dearnley ibid.

[475]Dearnaley D.P. op. cit. p. 24.

[476]Dearnaly D.P. et al op. cit. p. 24.

[477]David Hume, An Enquiry Concerning Human Understanding, IV as quoted by Wasley C. Salmon in The Foundations of Scientific Inference. University of Pittsburgh Press. p.1, 1967.

[478]Ivan Illych. Medical Nemesis.

[479]Druss B., Marcus S.C., Olfson M, Tanielian T., and Pincus H.H. Trends in care by non-physician clinicians in the United States. N Eg J Med 348: p. 130, 2003.

[480]Druss B. op. cit. p. 136.

[481]Aiken L.H. Achieving an interdisciplinary workforce in health care. N. Eng. J. Med. 348:p. 162, 2003.

[482]Candace B. Pert, Phd, Molecules of Emostion. Simone and Schuster. N.Y.C. 1997.

[483]"Our society focuses on the consumer, puts the consumer in the driver's seat. It is misleading to think that someone who doesn't do this day in and day out can understand the factors in making this kind of decision." – Charles Peters, M.D. quoted by A. D. Marcus in regard to bone marrow transplants in WSJ Teusday July 8th, 2003.

[484]I once volunteered to give a lecture to the clinic staff of one of my V.A.'s. In the lecture, I told them of a famous paper by J. Grayhack in the early 1950s which documented that not all men subjected to castration became impotent. For my trouble, namely telling them something of which they were unaware, something scholarly, I was denounced as "patriarchal" by one of the group who did not believe erections were possible after castration.

[485]Thomas Friedman, The Lexus and the Olive Tree.

[486]Janson T. A natural history of Latin. Oxford University Press. New York, 2004, p. 295.

[487]Lawrence Klotz, Re: The Prostate Cancer Prevention Trial…AUA News p. 13, Nov. 2007

[488]The Southwest Oncology Group advertised for patients in the Sept. 2004 Urology Times

[489]Zhang M., Atluwaijiri S., et al Vitamin E succinate inhibits human prostate cancer cell invasivenss and reduces the release of matrix metalloproteinases 85th Endocrine Society Meeting June 19-22, 2003 Philadelphia PA.

[490]The Western Section of the American Urological Association in October 28, 2008, in Monterey, California.

[491]Bankhead C. Soy derivative may lower PSA in PCa patients. Urology Times December 2003: p. 17.

[492]Pollard M. op. cit.

[493]Horan A.H. unpublished.

[494]Mulcahy M. quoting Ulf Tunn M.D. of Offenbach at the A.U.A. meeting. "Intermittent suppression as effective as continuous. Urology Times. Sept. 2004, p. 21.

[495]Astancolle S, Guidetti G, Pinna C, Corti A, Bettuzzi S. Increased levels of clusterin (SGP-2) mRNA and protein accompany rat ventral prostate involution following finasteride treatment. J. Endocrinol. 167: p. 197, 2000.

[496]James Eastman/Surgery and MSKCC.

[497]Urology Times 32(1) p. 20, 2004.

[498]Thomas Friedman, on Washington Week in Review.

[499]Horan A.H. The suppression of inflammatory edema at the nidation site by sodium salicylate and nitrogen mustard in the rat. Fert. and Steril. 22: 392, 1971.

[500]Pollack A. Drugs may turn cancer into manageable disease. N.Y.Times, June 6, 2004.

[501]Kaufman D.S. et al. A 63 year old man with metastatic prostate carcinoma refractory to hormone therapy. N. Eng. J. Med. 351: p. 171, 2004.

[502]Palkhivala A. "HIF U continues to show promise in early Pca" Urology Times 32(1)p. 1, 2004.

[503]Bankhead C. quoting M. Gleave M.D. Urology Times. Sept. 2004. p. 24.

[504]Mark Twain Tonight with Hal Holbrook.

[505]Guttman C. "Soy based supplement delays PSA progression." Urology Times. Sept. 2004, p. 21.

[506]Sheehan G. Going the Distance: One Man's Journey to the End of his Life. With an introduction by Robert Lypsite. Villard N.Y. New York 1996.

[507]Urology Times 32(1) p. 24, 2004.

[508]de Taille A., et al Prospective evaluation of a 21-sample needle biopsy procedure designed to improve the prostate cancer detection rate. Urology 61: p. 1181, 2003.

[509]Aix.1.uottowa.ca/-sulliv

[510]at a Western Section of the American Urological Association Thursday morning session on prostate cancer.

[511]The rules and definitions of treatment and outcome are decided upon and written before the clinical trial begins. There are no mid-course changes of treatment, timing of treatment, or changes in the definition of outcome.

[512]The treatment, or lack thereof, is chosen for the patient by the operations of chance alone as by flipping a coin or using a table of random numbers.

[513]Barron H. Lerner. The Breast Cancer Wars. Oxford University Press, New York: p. 225, 2001

[514]Middleton R.G. et al Prostate cancer clincical guidelines panel summary report on the management of clinically localized prostate cancer. J. Urol. 154: p. 2146, 1995.

[515]Stamey T.A. Editorial re "Introduction to Baysian Analysis" 1991 Monographs in Urology 12 (2) p. 17. Medical Directions Publishing Co. West Point PA.

516Steadman's medical dictionary, 26th Edition, 1995, p. 1642.

517Chang P. J. "Evaluating imaging test performance: an introduction to Bayesian analysis for urologists. 1991 Monographs in Urology 12 (2) p. 21. Medical Directions Publishing Co. West Point PA.

518P(D/T)=(TPR* Prior Prob) (TPR* Prior Prob) + (FPR*(1-Prior Prop)) "Bayes's theorem shows how the posterior probability (P(D/T+) represent the probability of having the disease if the disease is positive) is a function not only of test efficacy (as defined by the sensitivity and specificity) but also the prior probability. TPR=true positive rate or sensitivity; FPR=false positive rate or (1-specificity). Chang P.J. op. cit. p. 22.

519I simply assert this. I have not found anywhere a statement about what an acceptable specificity is. The reason is that what is acceptable is a line describing the releationship between sensitivity and specificity which bow sharply toward the corner where both values=1, and far from the diagonal between the points where both are zero.

CPSIA information can be obtained
at www.ICGtesting.com
Printed in the USA
BVHW060116020222
627784BV00005B/318

9 781641 119856